HORMONE RESET DIET 2 IN 1 VALUE BUNDLE

Hormone reset diet + Autophagy - #1 beginner's guide to lose weight + 21 days hormone-meal plans

Alexander Phenix

© Copyright 2019 - All rights reserved.

The content contained within this book may not be reproduced, duplicated, or transmitted without direct written permission from the author or the publisher.

Under no circumstances will any blame or legal responsibility be held against the publisher, or author, for any damages, reparation, or monetary loss due to the information contained within this book, either directly or indirectly.

Legal Notice:

This book is copyright protected. It is only for personal use. You cannot amend, distribute, sell, use, quote or paraphrase any part, or the content within this book, without the consent of the author or publisher.

Disclaimer Notice:

Please note the information contained within this document is for educational and entertainment purposes only. All effort has been executed to present accurate, up to date, reliable, complete information. No warranties of any kind are declared or implied. Readers acknowledge that the author is not engaging in the rendering of legal, financial, medical, or professional advice. The content within this book has been derived from various sources. Please consult a licensed professional before attempting any techniques outlined in this book.

By reading this document, the reader agrees that under no circumstances is the author responsible for any losses, direct or indirect, that are incurred as a result of the use of the information contained within this document, including, but not limited to, errors, omissions, or inaccuracies.

Table of Contents
HORMONE RESET DIET

Chapter 1: What is the Hormone Reset Diet? 2
   The 7 Hormones 5
   A 21-day Hormonal Reset 12
   More Than Just a Diet 15
Chapter 2: 21 Day Reset Preparation 20
   Adjust Your Eating Patterns 22
   Get Back to Nature.. 28
   Manage Your Stress 31
Chapter 3: Estrogen.. 37
   Balance Estrogen Levels with Food 41
   Additional Tips to Help Regulate Estrogen............. 46
Chapter 4: Insulin... 49
   Balance Insulin Levels with Food 53
   Additional Tips for Supporting Insulin 58
Chapter 5: Leptin.. 62
   Balance Leptin Levels with Food 66
   Additional Tips for Supporting Leptin 71
Chapter 6: Cortisol.. 75
   Balance Cortisol Levels with Food 79
   Additional Tips for Lowering Cortisol Levels.......... 83
Chapter 7: Thyroid Hormones 89
   Balance Thyroid Hormone with Food..................... 95
   Additional Tips for Healthy Thyroid Function...... 100
Chapter 8: Growth Hormone.................................. 104
   Balance Growth Hormone with Food 108
   Additional Tips for Naturally Regulating
   Growth Hormone... 113

Chapter 9: Testosterone 117
   Balance Testosterone with Food 122
   Additional Tips for Supporting Testosterone
   Levels 127
Chapter 10: What to do after Your Reset................134
   Gradually Reintegrate Food 135
   Adjust For Sensitivities and Intolerances..............139
   Focus on Quality 145
Chapter 11: Physical Fitness is Always Helpful 150
   Fitness During the 21-Day Diet 151
   Fitness after the 21-Day Diet................................155
   Find the Right Fitness for You 160
Conclusion 164
   An Effective Hormone Reset Diet 166
   Sustaining Hormone Health for Life 168
References 170
Appendix 1: Meal Planning 172
   Breakfast Scramble 173
   Buddha Bowls 177
   Super Soup..181
   Stuffed Veggies..184
   Spiced Chia Pudding 187

Table of Contents
AUTOPHAGY

Chapter 1: Here Are the Processes and Paths 190
   Types of Autophagy 198
Chapter 2: What Could These Benefits of Autophagy Be? 204
Chapter 3: Its Own Function 210
Chapter 4: How Can We Behave Better by Applying Intermittent Fasting? 221
   Benefits and Facts of Intermittent Fasting 233
Chapter 5: Here Is How to Set up a Good Keto Diet 246
Chapter 6: Let's Talk About Intermittent Fasting, but What Should We Drink? Here Are the Best Drinks 258
Chapter 7: How to Live a Healthy Life Thanks to the Constancy of Physical Exercise 266
Chapter 8: Let Us Immediately Set a New Mentality 284
Chapter 9: Autophagy Is the Possible New "Achilles Heel" Against Cancer 309
Chapter 10: Autophagy and Its Great Success 313
Conclusion 332
References 338

HORMONE RESET DIET

How to Learn the Basic 7 Hormone Diet Strategies with Results in Just 21 Days of Weight Loss and Metabolism Establishment

Alexander Phenix

Chapter 1:

What is the Hormone Reset Diet?

Understanding why this reset will work for you is an important part of the process to help you maintain your willpower and dedication throughout the next 21 days and beyond.

Hormones are responsible for much more than your teenager's mood swings and acne, or whether you'll be more likely to get pregnant in your 40s or start perimenopause.

We have over 50 different types of hormones that are responsible for regulating metabolism, sleep cycles, stress responses, growth rates of all kinds, and generally just keeping you alive by maintaining homeostasis in your body.

Your endocrine and nervous systems work together to send information throughout your body, triggered by both external factors, as well as need to keep the autonomic functions of your body operational at all times.

Your nervous system is lighting fast and transmits messages directly to cells for instant, short-lived responses. Your endocrine system, on the other hand, is more slow-moving, transmitting messages throughout your entire body using your blood.

Within your endocrine system, there is a collection of glands that make and secrete hormones. Some of these hormones do the work, and others delegate, simply acting as messengers telling another hormone what to do and when to do it.

Each hormone has a specific target cell type that it's able to communicate with through receptors on the cell. When a target cell is activated, the hormone either increases or decreases its function to keep your body homeostasis or balance.

If the receptors become damaged, the hormone can't effectively communicate with the cell, and processes inside of your body become confused and break down.

For women, there are seven hormones in particular that influence your metabolism and how your body decides to store or use energy. If these hormones fall out of balance, you'll be faced with weight gain and weight loss resistance, among many other frustrating and dangerous side-effects.

The 7 Hormones

If you can rebalance your hormones so that they're communicating with your cells and nervous system properly, your body will naturally regulate your weight. Humans are designed for efficiency, and holding on to unnecessary weight is anything but efficient.

The seven hormones we'll focus on throughout this 21-day reset are estrogen, insulin, leptin, cortisol, thyroid, growth, and testosterone.

Each hormone has its own chapter, which will explain in depth what proper function of the hormone should be like and how to get it back to normal. For now, let's take a quick look at the hormones you'll be working with.

Estrogen

Both men and women have estrogen, but it's particularly prevalent in women. It's responsible not only for a healthy reproductive system, but it also affects the heart and blood vessels, skin and hair production, and the health of your brain and bones.

Estrogen production is easily thrown out of order by our food and lifestyle choices, but high estrogen isn't the only problem. The key is to maintain a balance between estrogen and progesterone. As we age, our body naturally begins to produce less progesterone.

If estrogen levels are already high, the balance will just become more and more dysregulated over time.

An imbalance in your estrogen levels can not only lead to irregular menstrual cycles, but it is also closely linked to weight gain, particularly around the hips, thighs, and belly.

Insulin

Insulin is most well-known because of its role in diabetes. It's the hormone responsible for keeping blood glucose levels at a healthy balance, but, unfortunately, due to diet and lifestyle choices, insulin resistance or metabolic syndrome, has become one of the fastest-growing diseases on earth.

For many years, this condition was thought to be caused by obesity, but studies are starting to show that the reverse is actually true. Obesity is a symptom of insulin resistance. If you can rebalance your insulin levels by monitoring what you eat and when, you can stop your body from sending the signals to store more energy in fat, and start losing weight instead.

Leptin

Leptin is often called the hunger hormone because it's responsible for telling your brain when you have enough fat stored in your body to keep you safe and when you need to take in more energy.

If you have low body fat, your brain will throw out hunger signals to encourage you to find food. Unfortunately, if you have damaged leptin receptors, your brain will also continue to pump out hunger signals, whether you're actually in need of energy or not.

Hunger is very hard to ignore, and if your leptin levels are dysregulated, not only are you going to feel hungry constantly, but your body will also be actively trying to store any energy you consume as fat instead of using it immediately.

Cortisol

Cortisol is known as your stress hormone. When you've got too much on your plate and life is running you ragged, cortisol comes to the rescue...in a manner of speaking.

When your hormones are all well-balanced, and you're operating a relatively healthy body, cortisol helps to regulate your metabolism and immune response, among other important jobs.

When your stress response is triggered, cortisol is the hormone that shuts off operations of non-essential services. From your body's point of view, there's no point in worrying about digesting your food, keeping your ovaries healthy, or protecting your memory if your immediate survival is in jeopardy.

All your energy is diverted to systems that will keep you alive in the face of danger, such as your heart rate and getting enough blood and energy to your muscles.

This system is fantastic when you're actually in a life or death situation, but chronically elevated cortisol can lead to long-term digestive issues, immune disorders, mental health disorders, and much more.

Thyroid hormones

Thyroid hormones interact with a variety of other hormone pathways, and it's absolutely necessary to support a healthy metabolism. The thyroid hormone helps to regulate growth hormone, as well as your levels of progesterone, which all work together to regulate healthy body weight.

Genetic factors play a key role in thyroid hormone production; however, so does your gut health. Your thyroid is often targeted by autoimmune responses caused by what is commonly known as "leaky gut" syndrome.

When your immune system mistakes thyroid hormones for intruders, not only will inflammation and other immune responses start to create chronic damage in your body, but your thyroid hormones will also not be produced or received properly.

This can cause weight gain and retention, mood disorders, and a severe drop in energy levels, among other undesirable results.

Growth hormone

Growth hormone is responsible for stimulating the growth of nearly every tissue in your body, including your bones. With the right balance of this amazing hormone, you can actually grow your bones longer, instead of grinding them down over the years.

Of course, everything in this reset is focused on balance. While growth hormone is a good thing, too much of it can lead to fast growth and even enlarged extremities in extreme circumstances.

More common, especially in women, is the low production of growth hormone. In chronic conditions, this can lead to atrophied muscles and a decrease in bone density.

The growth hormone interacts with every other hormone your body produces. It helps to regulate the production of estrogen, insulin, and cortisol, and in turn, testosterone, leptin, and thyroid hormones keep growth hormone in check. Balance, on all accounts, is critical for overall healthy hormone function.

Similar to thyroid hormone, growth hormone is often mistaken for invasive proteins when your gut microbiome is in poor health. Autoimmune disorders caused by food sensitivities, particularly to dairy, in this case, can attack growth hormones, throwing your entire endocrine system out of sync.

Testosterone

Testosterone is a sex hormone that is found in higher concentrations in men but is still very important in women. Low levels have been linked to poor sex drive, but having too much can cause infertility.

It's not only concerned with your reproductive system, though. Testosterone helps to increase growth hormone and, together, they encourage lean muscle mass and fat burning. Without it, you can become resistant to weight loss, among other symptoms.

Men produce testosterone primarily in their testes, but women split the minute production between four different glands and tissues. This can be both good and bad. It helps to split the responsibility of maintaining the optimal balance between multiple players, but this can also cause a cascade of disruption between those same players.

As with all your hormones, balance is key.

A 21-day Hormonal Reset

Weight gain, fatigue, mood disorders, digestive struggles, and other uncomfortable *diseases* are your body's way of telling you something is wrong. It is not normal to feel unwell.

Many of these symptoms, especially for women, are signals that your endocrine system has a glitch. It isn't producing hormones effectively enough to manage your metabolism properly.

As we've already mentioned, the good news is that hormones are quick to reset themselves. Your body desperately wants to be in homeostasis, so if you can support its needs, it will gladly reset.

What a Reset Isn't

First and foremost, let's get clear on what a reset *isn't*.

A hormone reset isn't a cleanse. It's not a trendy detox or a quick fix.

It's not an easy button that will let you drop the last seven pounds so you can fit into your little black dress for one specific special occasion and then coast right back into your unhealthy habits.

A hormone reset isn't an overnight cure for metabolic diseases. For that matter, it isn't a *cure* for anything.

To be completely honest with you, this hormone reset isn't always going to be easy on you. You'll be asked to give up foods that you're chemically addicted to and some that you simply enjoy eating. You might experience symptoms of withdrawal, and some days you might feel worse before you start to feel better.

The next 21 days aren't all going to be pleasant. You'll be encouraged to support your dietary changes with lifestyle changes that might be out of your comfort zone right now.

But if you can commit to this hormone reset, and all its hard moments, by the end of it you will have naturally reset multiple systems in your body so that not only can you lose weight, but you'll also have more energy, better sleep, less stress and, overall, you'll get a lot more enjoyment out of the simple act of living each day.

What a Reset Is

It takes about 72 hours to clean your blood of excess hormones and bring it back into balance, so every three days of this reset, you'll be focused on a single hormone.

For the next three weeks, you'll systematically eliminate foods that are known to disrupt hormone production, and you'll add in foods that have been shown to help support your hormone production.

By resetting the hormones that are primarily responsible for your metabolism, you'll be able to finally coax your body into releasing any weight that is unnecessary—like those last seven pounds!

The best part of bringing your hormones back into balance is that when everything in your body is communicating clearly and all systems are operating well, you'll no longer be getting mixed signals from your body.

You'll get hungry when you need more energy, not when you're bored or emotional. You'll crave foods that make you feel alive, young, and energetic, and you'll have no trouble saying "no" to the heavy, bloating, guilt-inducing snacks of your past.

More Than Just a Diet

Studies have shown that weight loss, especially in women, is more effective when you control what you eat than when you focus on exercise. While there is some truth to the relationship between calories consumed and calories burned, contributing to weight gain, there is a lot more going on inside your body than simple mathematics. The quality of the calories you consume can be just as important as the quantity.

That's why this diet doesn't focus on numbers, but rather on the type of food you're eating, how you're eating it, and what your eating patterns are telling your body.

This type of diet can be supplemented by vitamins, but, more importantly, it can be supplemented by your mind and your movement.

Mindset

Editing your eating plan to become healthier and support balanced hormones isn't all about what you can't eat. It's just as much about what can eat and should be eating more of.

In cognitive-behavioral therapy, how a person *thinks* about a situation has a massive impact on how that person feels and reacts to that situation.

In other words, how you think about the food on your plate can have a greater effect on the way you enjoy it than the taste of the food itself. If you start this program focused on everything you have to give up, you'll make it impossible for yourself to appreciate all the incredible foods you're welcome to eat.

Instead, if you pay attention to the variety of flavors and beauty of the foods that you're encouraged to eat in abundance, you'll find yourself spoilt for choice throughout this program.

To help you keep a positive mindset throughout this process, and remind you why you've chosen to reset your hormones, you might find it useful to keep a journal.

You can use your journal to track your emotional ups and downs through the process, as well as your physical changes. Keeping track of your progress is a great way to stay motivated and determined to continue.

Make a note of how you feel before and after

each hormonal reset, and any major changes you notice. While it may sound gross, you can even track your bathroom habits, making a note of how you digest different foods.

Throughout the next 21 days, you will be tempted to give up at some point. Having a really great reason to continue, and a few reminders of your progress might be the deciding factor in your desire to continue toward resetting your health.

You and your future health are worth it.

Physical Activity

As previously mentioned, your secret to losing weight is mainly dependent on the foods you're eating. But that doesn't mean exercise won't factor into the next 21 days at all.

Think of physical activity as a supporting role in your health. Without it, your results will be limited but, more importantly, if exercise isn't a part of your daily life, your long term health is guaranteed to suffer.

Luckily, the first few days of the reset will take exercise nice and easy, and the remainder of the program will be a slow yet steady intensity increase. The best news is that, if you follow the fitness tips recommended in Chapter 11, you won't be running for miles on end or spending hours upon hours in the gym. Instead, you'll be exercising more effectively to not only support weight loss but to make sure you keep the weight off long term and support healthy lean muscle and bone density for the rest of your life.

If you've taken the advice to start a hormone reset journal, you'll want to take a few key measurements before you get started so that in the end, you know exactly how far you've come.

Using a flexible measuring tape, jot down your measurements around your bust, waist, and at the fullest part of your hips and butt. If you tend to carry a lot of your weight in the lower half of your body, you can also measure each thigh. Similarly, if you're concerned about your arms, you can measure your biceps.

Of course, you'll also want to record your starting weight. It's a good idea to step on the scale first thing in the morning and just before bed the day before you start the reset.

By the end of the 21 days, your weight shouldn't fluctuate as drastically throughout the day, but before you begin, you could have a variance of five pounds or even more. It will be interesting to see how this fluctuation improves over time.

It's also a good idea to track physical symptoms like soreness, inflammation, headaches, etc. Ideally, over the next few weeks, you'll notice a steady improvement, but there may be times when the reset makes you feel worse before it makes you feel better. Making a note of any changes along the way can be motivating and enlightening.

The more you learn about your body now, the more power you'll have in the future to make tweaks to your lifestyle in the name of health.

Chapter 2:

21 Day Reset Preparation

The first and perhaps most important step in this process is to consult with your doctor or a nutritionist or dietician who is familiar with any current health concerns you may have. They will be able to provide more in-depth and personalized information, as well as answer any questions that might come up for you as you work your way through the reset.

If you don't have any preexisting conditions or a doctor that you see regularly, you may want to consider working with an integrative physician in your area. An integrative doctor is not only trained in conventional allopathic medicine but also understands and respects the body's natural ability to heal itself without prescription medications.

Working with a professional will help you fill in any micro-nutrient gaps you may have. Understand that it's very difficult to get 100% of the nutrition your body needs to truly thrive from food, both because of a lack of knowledge about what you need as well as a lack of availability.

You're probably incredibly effective at your trained profession, but if you're not an expert in hormone health, nutrition, physical fitness, *and* the intricate workings of the human body–that's okay!

Even if you knew everything about nutrition, there is to know, and you still might need to supplement it. Soil and produce quality are not what they used to be, not to mention location-based quality and availability.

With each hormone reset, you'll learn the most important vitamins and nutrients to support your hormone function, and if you feel the need to supplement, you'll have the option to do so.

From here on out, try not to obsess too much about every last detail. The more you focus on getting everything absolutely perfect, the more stressed you're going to get. As will become very apparent as you work your way through this book, stress is the enemy your hormones! Do what you can to the best of your ability, and let the rest take care of itself.

Nobody's perfect.

Adjust Your Eating Patterns

One of the reasons many women find following a strict diet helpful is because it tells you exactly what to eat, what not to eat, how much to eat, and sometimes even when to eat. Following orders for a short, set period of time leaves no room for mistakes.

But what happens when you go back to "real life?" Without the rigid structure of your diet, you fall right back into your old ways, and all the weight and disorders come right back.

With the 21 day reset, you'll have guidelines to help you understand what to eat and what to avoid, but it's not as restrictive as a standard caloric diet, and it naturally helps reset your eating patterns while it's working toward resetting your hormones.

By following this reset, you'll be establishing a new relationship with your meals. These new eating patterns will be easy to maintain long-term once you've developed a habit, helping to ensure your results are also long-term.

Respect Mealtime

While you do the reset, it's important that you

practice structured mealtimes. Your hormones and nearly every other biological system in your body thrive off of routine.

By committing to three regular meals a day, eaten at relatively the same time each day, you'll be sending your body the message that it can expect to refuel at certain times, and there's no need to panic and start storing fat overnight.

On the other hand, if you train your body to expect food every two hours by constant grazing and snacking, it will want to be fed every two hours. Not only is this inconvenient, but it's also unsafe and dangerous to your health.

Digesting food is a lot of hard work, and your body needs time to get it done. Leaving 4 - 6 hours between meals and a minimum of 12 hours of overnight fasting will help your digestion keep up with its workload and run more smoothly.

You can also think about it this way: if you want your body to start burning fat, you have to give it the opportunity to do so. You need to stop eating all the time!

This is not just to reduce the availability of energy in the form of calories, but it's crucial to the regulation of hormones that tell your body when to store energy for times of need and when to *use* that stored energy.

Eat Real Food

One of the best things you can do for your overall health and certainly help rebalance your hormones is to move away from packages and toward whole foods, as close to their natural state as possible.

Throughout the 21 days reset, you'll focus on certain foods every three days, both to eliminate as well as to add. As a universal rule, you want to avoid processed, packaged, and pre-prepared foods as much as possible.

If you're budget and location allows, it's also important to choose organic foods to cook with. When it comes to meat, eggs, and dairy, choosing organic pasture-fed and finished, will make sure you're not ingesting a host of synthetic hormones that will mess up your progress.

Organic produce will protect you from hormone-disrupting toxins so, at the very least, have a look at the current "dirty dozen" and pick organic, local, and seasonal produce at every opportunity.

When you're grocery shopping, don't be fooled by marketing. Keep in mind that the food industry is a very lucrative business, but it is a business. Food producers want you to buy their food, and they'll say just about anything to trick you into eating more of what they have to offer. Just because something says, "natural" or "heart-healthy" doesn't mean it is.

When you cook from scratch, using whole food ingredients, you know exactly what you're eating, and you're eating in the way nature intended. Macronutrients, micronutrients, and fiber all work together in harmony when you eat whole foods rather than broken down, isolated pieces of food made in a laboratory somewhere.

Before you even get started, it's helpful to know and admit to your weaknesses. Create a chart for yourself that predicts which foods are going to call out to you when you're having a particularly rough day.

Create a "swap chart" for yourself. Identify foods that you constantly crave even though you know they aren't a part of a healthy diet. For example, your chart might have a column that lists ice cream, cookies, potato chips, fried chicken, and fast food.

Next to each of your weaknesses, write down a few options for swaps that you'll eat instead. Berries instead of cookies, popcorn instead of chips, and homemade, healthy freezer meals instead of fast food.

When you have an immediate and easily available alternative, you'll be much better prepared to avoid potential pitfalls.

Get in the Habit of Cooking

If you're buying real food for yourself and your family, you're going to have to get into the habit of cooking. A lot of people worry that cooking is too time-consuming, but with practice and strategy, home cooking can be faster and less expensive than eating out.

As with anything in life, the more you practice, the better you'll become.

Batch cooking and freezing food is one great strategy to implement. It's almost always more cost-effective to work in bulk, and cooking a larger batch of food doesn't often take much longer than cooking up a single serving.

You'll not only save time and money in the long run, but you'll be taking the guesswork and stress out of what to eat when time isn't on your side. Whenever you run up against a deadline, or feel under the weather or don't have time to cook for any other reason, instead of finding yourself tipping a delivery driver, all you'll have to do is take a look in your freezer.

Cooking itself can become a stress-relieving activity, bringing its own sense of joy an accomplishment to the table. Eating a delicious meal that you prepared is satisfying and something you can be proud of.

Spending more time hustling around your kitchen even adds up to more physical activity when compared to the alternative of sitting in your car as you go through a drive-thru. It may seem minor to you right now, but every minute you spend moving around instead of sitting has a dramatic impact on your hormonal health.

To help you flex your new cooking muscles, there is a collection of meal ideas at the back of the book to get you started. From breakfast, lunch, dinner, and even dessert, you'll have plenty of inspiration to get you through the next 21 days and well beyond.

Be prepared; these aren't recipes, but more like guides to helping you create your own unique recipes.

Get Back to Nature

Human bodies were not designed to spend 16 hours a day seated and another eight lying down.

They are pretty spectacular, though. As nature intended, our biological systems are self-healing, self-detoxifying, and designed to coordinate multiple systems in perfect harmony.

Unfortunately, because of our large and advanced capacity to think, human advancement has allowed us to deviate from nature in many ways.

We discovered how to modify and influence nearly every aspect of the human condition, from what we eat to how we sleep and move.

Just because we can process and modified foods to make them addictingly more palatable doesn't mean we should. Just because light bulbs and screens make it possible for us to lengthen our days and alter our sleeping patterns at will, doesn't make it healthy to do so. Finally, just because we don't have to chase our food down in a primeval hunt doesn't mean we don't need to find another way to move our bodies.

If you want to improve your health, one of the best things you can do is return to nature.

Circadian Rhythms

By definition, a circadian rhythm is "a natural, internal process that regulates the sleep-wake cycle and repeats roughly every 24 hours ("Circadian rhythm," n.d.)."

Following natural sleep patterns based on the rising and setting sun and regularized bedtimes allow you to spend more quality time in a deep sleep. Among other benefits, deep sleep increases the production of growth hormone, which, as you'll learn in Chapter 8, helps to regulate weight, particularly belly fat.

While you're on the Hormone Reset Diet, it's important to give your body as much opportunity to heal as possible. This means getting a minimum of eight hours of sleep every day and, if possible, up to 10 hours.

It can be very informative to keep your journal by your bed and make notes before you go to sleep, and when you wake up. Track the quality of your sleep, how well-rested you feel, how long it takes you to fall asleep, how tired you are at bedtime, stress levels, and general feelings at the end of the day and the beginning of a new day.

As you work your way through the 21 days, all of these metrics should start to improve.

The Great Outdoors

Unless you live in the middle of a highly polluted city, taking time each day to spend at least a half-hour outdoors every day can help reestablish the balance between serotonin and cortisol. Exposure to fresh air and sunshine gives you the opportunity to benefit from nature's ability to help you relax and get in a better mood.

Not all nutrients are taken in through food. Some are absorbed through your skin and from the air you breathe. Going for a walk in an area with plenty of trees improves the air quality and stimulates mental functions that can help protect your brain from cognitive decline.

When you get out into nature, use it as an excuse to unplug, leaving all your electronics at home. The physical movement, natural environment, and lack of immediate responsibilities will help you unwind. Focus on your breathing, find your own personal style of mediation, and simply appreciate the good things in life.

The boost of Vitamin D and oxygen helps to regulate your hormones and many other aspects of your overall health as well.

As little as 10 minutes can make a noticeable difference in your mood and energy levels, but dedicating 30 minutes a day to spend outdoors is ideal.

Manage Your Stress

Stress is getting blamed for just about every health disorder we can identify, and yet very little is being done actually to change or eliminate what causes us stress.

When it comes to stress and relaxation, sometimes the smallest things can make the biggest difference. You may not be able to quit your job, overcome your financial woes, or find yourself in the midst of the perfect family life, but you *can* work on your breath and meditation.

Both of these techniques are extremely powerful at reducing stress levels and, conveniently, they're both free, simple, can be done anywhere, at nearly any time, and only take a few minutes of your time.

There will be an entire chapter dedicated to cortisol, which is the hormone most closely related to stress. To help you prepare for this chapter, you should know upfront that you will be encouraged to eliminate caffeine from your diet during this reset completely. If you drink a lot of coffee, it is more than likely adding to your stress levels. It's a good idea to start reducing your consumption now, in preparation for Chapter 6, which begins on day 10 of your reset.

A good way to reduce reliance on caffeine progressively is to start cutting back and making strategic swaps at the same time. Depending on how many caffeinated beverages you drink daily now, try cutting that number in half, starting today.

Because sugar is just as addictive as caffeine, you'll also want to reduce the amount of sweetener you use in your coffee or tea. By the time you get to the cortisol reset, you will have already reduced or eliminated sugar, so removing caffeine should be much easier than you expect.

Every time you would normally reach for a cup of coffee or tea, replace it with decaf, green tea, or glass of water half the time. This will help you hydrate as well, which is a simple, non-hormonal way to keep your energy levels elevated.

On days three to five of the reset, try replacing all of your coffee with decaf and all your black tea with green tea or, even better, green tea.

For days six through eight, try to consume only green tea and non-caffeinated beverages. By day 10, you should be ready to wean yourself off of coffee completely.

Finally, exercise is a key component to relieving stress, though it isn't the main focus of this reset. You should start incorporating movement into your days on a regular basis if you're not already. Chapter 11 covers recommended fitness efforts during the reset as well as after the reset and for the rest of your life. It might be helpful to read through that chapter before you start the program.

Breath Work

When you're in a state of stress, your body increases your heart rate, breathing rate, and blood pressure to give your muscles and brain the exact resources it needs to cleverly and speedily save your life.

The primary reason you breath is to absorb oxygen and remove carbon dioxide from your body. When you're stressed, you are more likely to take shallow breaths to get more oxygen into your body to aerobic power activity, like running for your life.

In nature's point of view, you cannot outrun a predator if you're taking deep, measured breaths. With that in mind, it should make sense that breathing deeply and calmly is a very effective "off" button for your stress response.

Breathing exercises help your parasympathetic system take over for your stressed sympathetic nervous system, reducing levels of cortisol in your blood, slowing your heart rate, and lowering your blood pressure, all thanks to a few deep, measured, and purposeful breaths.

Using breath work to reduce stress is that it only takes a few minutes, can be done anywhere by anyone, and it's completely free.

Meditation

Most people fall into one of two camps when it comes to meditation: you either love it or you hate it. Before you dismiss this section outright, try to understand the simplicity and the benefits of taking up this practice.

Meditation either uses negation or focus techniques.

The goal of negation is to clear your mind, leaving it blank. This allows you to release all of your cares and worries for at least a few minutes, giving you space to breathe easier and relax. When accomplished effectively, it can leave you in a state of semi-consciousness or even unconsciousness, similar to sleeping. If you can get to this point, you give your brain a chance to recover.

On the other side of the spectrum, focus techniques encourage you to devote all of your attention to a single thought, feeling, or purpose. If you can master this technique, you will be better able to avoid distractions in all areas of your life.

Focus, for most people, is much easier to achieve than clearly your mind completely, and it can be used as a stepping stone for the more advanced negation practice.

If you have been finding that stress in your life is causing exhaustion during the day, when you need to be busy at work, which compounds your feeling of stress, a few minutes dedicated to focus will help you relax and pull your attention back to the task at hand. It stimulates wakefulness and can help you feel re-energized.

If stress is having a bigger effect on your sleeping patterns, a few minutes of guided meditations to help you clear your mind and leave the day behind you can help you get better sleep, improving your health in many ways.

Regardless of what kind of meditation you try, give yourself permission to be terrible at first. It's a skill that needs to be honed over time, but in just a few minutes a day, you should see noticeable improvements within a few weeks.

Chapter 3:

Estrogen

Estrogen is well-known as the hormone that gives a woman her feminine shape by filling out breasts and hips, but it triggers many other responses in the body as well.

We've talked about how important homeostasis is to health, and when it comes to estrogen, the ideal balance is found in a relationship with its hormonal partner, progesterone.

For instance, during a woman's menstrual cycle, estrogen is responsible for the growth of the uterine lining, whereas progesterone helps release it at the end of the cycle. They need to work together to ensure a complete, safe, and healthy cycle.

Cycles are a common theme in healthy biological systems. Along with balance, your hormones are very particular in the way they are used. For some processes occurring in your body, recycling is a great thing. Taking broken components of dead or damaged cells and turning them into healthy building blocks for new cells is what keeps your body youthful and in good working order.

Estrogen, however, is not meant to be recycled. Once it's produced, it's meant to be used as intended and then removed from your body.

Estrogen Dominance and Pollution

For most women, by the time you hit your 30s, your body starts to produce less progesterone, leading to estrogen dominance. To compound the problem, certain other hormones can upset the balance even further. Cortisol, for example, can block progesterone receptors, causing the ratio of estrogen to progesterone to lurch even further out of sync.

Not producing enough progesterone is only one-way balance is disrupted. A diet heavy in estrogen-laden foods, a stressful lifestyle, and a digestive system that doesn't effectively remove used up hormones and waste can also lead to disruptions.

Estrogen pollution is just what it sounds like—a build-up of estrogen that turns a healthy, essential hormone into a pollutant due to excess. Estrogen dominance and pollution is a long-term problem that doesn't happen overnight or because your balance is thrown off during one particularly stressful day.

When you've had too much estrogen coursing through your blood for too long, it can lead to weight gain, obesity, and cancer.

Doctors trained in the conventional medical system are taught to prescribe birth control medication to women under 50 who have any disorder that might be connected to an issue with estrogen. The added synthetic progesterone helps to balance out the estrogen.

After 50, women are assumed to be showing symptoms of menopause and will instead be prescribed hormone replacement therapy.

There may be a place and a time for prescription medications, but neither of these solutions actually *heal* your body, they simply mask your symptoms. A dietary reset can help balance your hormones naturally without a cascade of side effects.

Symptoms and Risks of Estrogen Dominance

If you've ever experienced breast tenderness or heavy, painful periods, your body has given you warning signs that your estrogen levels are getting too dominant.

PMS and mood issues are talked about as if they're a normal experience of being a woman, but, in reality, these are symptoms as well. Nothing about being in pain or discomfort should ever be considered *normal.*

If you'd like more scientific data about your own personal estrogen levels, getting regular PAP smears will help you, and your doctor notices any changes that happen over time.

Unfortunately, moodiness and sore breasts are minor symptoms of dysregulated hormones, but the development of cysts, resistance to weight loss, endometriosis, and even cancer are more severe and equally common symptoms.

Nobody likes to talk about breast cancer, but most women around the world live in fear of it. It's not a causeless fear, either. According to US statistics, one in eight American women will develop an invasive form of the disease at some point in her life (BreastCancer.org, 2019). If you balance your estrogen levels, you can play a part in decreasing that statistic by at least one woman.

Having too much estrogen floating around in your body is not a condition you want to take

Alcohol raises estrogen levels, and there's no good way to sugarcoat this fact. If you're struggling with your estrogen levels, alcohol will add to the problem.

It also slows down metabolism, further disrupts your astrobleme, raises cortisol levels, which, as we know, further disrupts your progesterone levels, and it challenges your sleep quality.

Your liver is a huge player when it comes to directing hormones through your bloodstream, and you probably won't be surprised to hear this, alcohol consumption wreaks havoc on your liver function.

Once your hormones are rebalanced, enjoying the occasional drink will not be overly detrimental to your health, but for the duration of this program, you'll want to avoid alcohol completely.

There is a very good chance that you'll feel and see a difference in your body within the first 72 hours of this plan, but it's crucial to keep the next 21 days free of all red meat and alcohol to really give your body a chance to recover. While estrogen might reset in three days, changing the flora in your gut takes longer but will be very beneficial to your overall success with this reset and your long-term health.

What to Enjoy More of

Since you won't be eating red meats like beef or pork, it's important to integrate alternative, clean proteins into your daily diet to keep your energy levels up. Some great sources of protein that will support healthy estrogen removal include:

- pastured poultry and eggs
- wild-caught, cold-water fish, especially salmon and sardines
- plant-based proteins such as quinoa, soy, buckwheat, legumes, nuts, seeds, especially chia & hemp seeds, and even algae like spirulina or chlorella

Finding the perfect balance of Omega 3 and Omega 6 fatty acids can help regulate your weight. A Standard American Diet (SAD) is disproportionately high in Omega 6s. By substituting processed food for salmon, sardines, and grass-fed butter, which are rich in Omega 3s, you'll be priming your body to burn fat instead of holding onto it.

Fiber is absolutely essential in helping your body remove waste. Studies have shown that 95% of Americans are deficient in this nutrient, which can lead to significant digestive issues, not to mention hormonal imbalances and a host of other chronic and life-threatening diseases (Quagliani & Felt-Gunderson, 2017).

Fiber-rich foods can help relieve symptoms of bloating and constipation and get rid of excess estrogen in the process.

Too much fiber all at once can be hard on your system, though, so increase your consumption gradually, adding 5 g a day until you reach an average of 45 g per day.

It's surprisingly easy to increase fiber in your diet as it's present in all plant-based foods. Some of the highest quality sources include:

- chia, ground flaxseed, lentils, legumes, berries, and green veggies

All vegetables have fiber, but they're also incredibly nutrient-dense, providing your body with vitamins, minerals, and antioxidants it needs to stay healthy overall. For estrogen balance focus on getting great variety in the colors of your vegetables:

- leafy greens, broccoli, carrots, bell peppers, cauliflower, squash

Additional Tips to Help Regulate Estrogen

For some reason, a great many man-made chemicals and additives shift the natural balance of estrogen in our systems because they mimic the effects of this particular hormone. There are over 700 synthetic chemicals that we run into on a daily basis that disrupt our estrogen production.

A lot of these chemicals aren't necessarily in our food, but they're in our skincare products, our household items, in the water we drink and the air we breathe. We go more in-depth on toxin-related disruption in Chapter 9.

By doing our best to eliminate synthetic hormones through our diet and support the normal function of our endocrine system, our bodies will be better able to handle the overload from outside influencers.

A Note about Soy

One of the food items that comes under a lot of scrutinies for mimicking the effects of estrogen in our systems is soy.

There are those who very passionately argue against soy, citing studies that show how it is a major contributor to the increase in estrogen dominance related disorders and diseases.

And then there are others who reference studies done on Asian cultures, where soy-based products are consumed in high quantities even though estrogen-related disorders are extremely low.

For the purposes of this Hormone Reset Diet, soy can be consumed in moderate quantities, but the focus should always be on quality.

What some of the studies in the anti-soy groups fail to mention is that isolated soy compounds are heavily used in processed foods, such as protein powders, textured soy protein, and processed meat alternatives.

Another issue is that the vast majority of soy consumed is eaten by animals in conventional industrial farms. One of the reasons soy products are contributing to estrogen dominance is not because humans are eating too much soy, but because we're eating too much animal protein, which is consuming too much soy.

If you eliminate processed foods and conventionally raised meat from your eating plan, you'll not only significantly decrease the amount of soy you eat, but you'll also be automatically decreasing the amount of sugar, gluten, unhealthy fats, and synthetic hormones that you're consuming as well.

Finally, when you're eating foods in their whole form, as opposed to isolating specific compounds, you provide your body with more nutritional support to effectively digest and process the food.

If you choose to eat soy products, choose non-GMO organic options that go through as little processing as possible. Organic edamame, tofu, and tempeh are fantastic sources of clean, plant-based proteins, packed with vitamins and minerals that will help your endocrine system thrive.

Chapter 4:

Insulin

Your metabolic system relies almost exclusively on glucose to provide energy to all your major biological systems and organs. On the surface, this may sound like you have to provide your body with glucose in order to function continuously, but that is far from the whole truth.

In a healthy, perfectly balanced body, blood glucose levels hold steady at about 70 - 100 mg/dL. Carbohydrates are the easiest macronutrient for your body to break down into glucose. When you eat carbs, your metabolic system has easy access to glucose, which raises your blood sugar levels.

Understanding Insulin

When glucose in your blood increases, beta cells in your pancreas produce and release insulin. Insulin is the almighty hormone responsible for telling your body to move glucose out of your bloodstream and into your adipose tissue for storage.

Before you start to blame every ounce of unwanted fat on insulin, it's important to recognize how important insulin is to your very survival. When blood sugar is chronically elevated, it can damage blood vessels, particularly those in your nervous system, heart, kidneys, eyes, and extremities, like your hands and feet.

Insulin is designed to protect against this kind of damage, while at the same time creating a backup plan for your future in case there comes a time when food is scarce.

Once enough, glucose has been moved out of your blood. Insulin production will shut down. If you don't reintroduce more food for an extended period of time, your blood sugar will continue to drop as your metabolic system continues to draw on that blood glucose for energy to maintain the normal operation.

If your blood sugar levels get too low, alpha cells in your pancreas trigger the production of glucagon, which tells your liver and adipose tissue to release the stored glucose back into your bloodstream.

If you continue to add new sources of glucose, however, your body will never need to tap into its stored energy and will instead continue to add to it with every new feeding.

Mediating Insulin Resistance

If your blood sugar levels are always high because you're constantly adding more glucose to your blood with constant snacking and grazing habits, your pancreas will be overworked, producing insulin to deal with the problem. At some point, there will simply be too much demand for insulin to keep up with, and your pancreas will start to fail.

Compounding this issue is the fact that if insulin is triggered too often, your body will stop responding to it properly. Sort of like the boy who called wolf, this is called insulin resistance, and if left unchecked can lead to Type 2 diabetes as well as a host of other health issues and consistent weight gain.

By regulating what you're eating and when, you can help support your body's normal insulin function, reestablishing the homeostatic relationship between insulin and glucagon.

Having too much insulin circulating in your bloodstream will also cause an increase in estrogen, which you learned about in the last chapter. This cascading effect can also lead to leptin resistance and a decrease in testosterone. Together, this combination of dysregulated hormones causes damage all over your body, steadily increases the amount of weight you gain, and is biologically incapable of losing.

Type 1 diabetes is not caused by diet or eating patterns, but rather it's a result of an underperforming pancreas. The pancreas simply does not produce enough insulin to regulate blood sugar properly and must be supplemented by externally administered insulin. Even with this in mind, choosing what and when you eat with care for your blood sugar levels can help regulate the disease more naturally though, to date, there is no cure for Type 1 diabetes, dietary or otherwise.

Balance Insulin Levels with Food

For many years, it was assumed that eating fat was the main reason for gaining fat. It's now understood that the problem is not with the fat you eat, but rather the sugar. When you're insulin resistant, your body stores glucose in fat cells, causing you to gain weight. To lose weight then, it makes sense that you'll want to eat less high-glucose foods.

Simple carbohydrates convert almost immediately to sugar in your bloodstream, and, of course, so does plain and simple sugar.

Your goal is to balance your eating plan and focus on dense nutrient options. If you severely restrict or eliminate all carbs from your diet, you can actually increase the production of reverse T3, which is the inactive form of thyroid hormone that blocks hormone receptors. You'll learn more about this in Chapter 8, but for now, suffice it to say some carbs are essential to your overall health.

At this stage in the reset, you want to pay attention to incorporating high-quality, healthy fats, clean proteins, and complex, slow metabolizing carbohydrates.

If you're planning on counting your carbs, keep in mind the fact that fiber, while considered a carbohydrate, actually passes through your digestive system without breaking down, so it isn't used as energy or raise blood glucose. When you look at the nutrition of a food item, net carbs are what will affect your blood sugar. To calculate net carbs, simply subtract the grams of fiber from the total carbohydrate count.

What to Eliminate and Avoid

Using the Glycemic Index (GI) to choose the food you eat is a useful way to understand how your food is going to affect your insulin levels.

High GI foods will convert to glucose more quickly, causing a corresponding spike in your insulin. Low GI foods take longer to break down and will have a more sustained effect on your insulin, without the undesirable spike and crash.

For the next three days, you're going to want to avoid foods that have a GI higher than 70. Some examples that are common in SAD include, but are not limited to:

- all added sugar and sweeteners, including white and cane sugar, honey, maple or corn syrup, and agave

- sugary drinks, including soda, energy drinks, sweet teas, and most fruit juices or punches

- Processed sweets like candy, cookies, chocolate bars, donuts, etc.

- white and whole wheat pieces of bread

- white rice, rice milk, and rice-based snacks like rice crackers

- sugared and processed breakfast cereals

- some fruits, particularly watermelon and very ripe bananas

- instant or boiled potatoes

Condiments and spreads like ketchup, bbq sauce, relish, and jam may show up as low or medium GI foods, but they are easy to eat in larger quantities than recommended, so be very conscious of your consumption of any pre-packaged sauces, dips, dressings or spreads.

When you're trying to decide what to swap your favorite soda or sweet treat for, don't assume you're making a healthy choice by opting for a sugar-free version. Artificial sweeteners can overstimulate your taste buds, making you even more attracted to sugary foods and causing you to find non-sweet foods distasteful. This is not natural and can lead to extremely disordered eating.

What to Enjoy More of

Slow releasing carbs are low on the glycemic index and generally come from whole food sources like plants that are also high in fiber. There are two types of fiber, and understanding the difference between soluble and insoluble fiber will take you one step closer to really understanding how your body processes the food you eat.

The soluble fiber, in its natural, unprocessed state, assists in the moderation of blood glucose levels. When it enters your digestive system and gets mixed with water, it thickens, becomes jelly-like, and sticks to the inside walls of your intestines.

The purpose of this is to slow your food down in the gastrointestinal tract, giving your digestive system more time to break it down into nutrients for use. This is why foods with high soluble fiber are lower on the GI because they take longer to convert to glucose.

Food choices that are high in soluble fiber and have low glycemic loads include:

- most fruits and vegetables, including avocados, pears, and stone fruits, Brussel sprouts, sweet potatoes, broccoli, and carrots

- legumes, such as black beans, kidney beans

- nuts and seeds, like flaxseeds, sunflower seeds, and hazelnuts

- some whole grains, particularly barley and oats

Insoluble fiber, on the other hand, doesn't slow food digestion. Instead, it adds bulk and weight to undigested waste, helping it move out of your intestines more efficiently, preventing constipation. It also helps to support the development of healthy bacteria in your gut microbiome, which has many benefits, both related and separate, to balanced hormones.

Insoluble fiber doesn't affect blood glucose levels, so even though it's great for digestion and health, it isn't as good of an indicator for food choices to regulate insulin specifically.

Additional Tips for Supporting Insulin

The more carbs you eat, and the more frequently throughout the day you eat them, regardless of quantity, the less likely your body will be to dip into its back up reserves. If weight loss is one of your goals, you want your body using the energy that is stored in your fat cells.

Some carbohydrates are necessary for health, but you're likely eating many more carbs than you realize at the expense of other important macronutrients like healthy fats and proteins. The most effective secret to reducing carbohydrates is to focus on eating whole foods and avoiding processed foods as much as possible, which is easier said than done, especially if you're dealing with a sugar addiction or are used to existing primarily off of premade foods.

Conquer Sugar Addiction

As with most addictions, a big part of overcoming your addiction is mindset and willpower. You must have a powerful reason for making a choice to "get sober" and stick to this commitment throughout all the withdrawal symptoms.

Sugar addiction is every bit as controlling as drug addiction. Sugar triggers a dopamine response, which is your body's natural way of providing you with a pleasant high for doing a good job at something. Unfortunately, the more sugar you eat, the more dysregulated your dopamine communication becomes, requiring a bigger "hit" to produce the same response.

Even if you don't consider yourself a sugar addict, if you've been eating a Standard American Diet for a significant amount of time, you're likely more dependent on your sugar high than you realize, thanks to the prevalence of simple carbs that convert quickly to glucose– like bread, pasta, and almost anything processed, sweet or not.

You'll need a strong mindset and a deep level of determination to kick this particular habit, but once you do, you will find that you feel great. You'll have more energy than you have in years, and you won't find yourself crashing nearly as often.

Get Comfortable in Your Kitchen

One of the best ways to clean up your carb intake is to start preparing your own meals from real, whole ingredients.

Almost everything that comes in a shelf-stable package has been tampered with in some way to make the food not only last longer but taste better. It's in the best interest of the food industry to get people addicted to eating. That's the best way to ensure they'll keep coming back for more, after all.

If you start cooking for yourself, you'll learn what foods are supposed to taste like, and your body will start processing them as nature intended.

Your taste buds play a significant role in your diet and your ability to maintain a healthy eating plan. It's normal to want to eat more food that tastes great and less food that you don't like.

What you might not realize, however, is that your taste buds could be lying to you.

A diet high in processed sugars, salts, and fats can damage your taste buds. They lose the ability to enjoy flavors that are healthy, getting confused by chemicals and additives.

Luckily, it doesn't take long to get your taste buds back to normal, and you can learn to like a wide variety of foods and flavors that you thought you would hate for life. To help this process along, you can try coaxing natural sugars out of vegetables by roasting them or adding healthy fats like olive oil or organic, pasture-fed butter.

By doing your own cooking, you'll develop a new relationship and respect for the food you eat, helping you adjust your mind as well as your hormones.

Chapter 5:

Leptin

Biologically speaking, the reason humans eat is to provide the body with the resources it requires to produce energy and keep all systems running efficiently. Under ideal circumstances, when you have enough power, you'll feel full. When you lack energy, your body will send out hunger signals to encourage you to eat again.

Unfortunately, for many different reasons, our bodies are rarely operating under ideal circumstances. For most of us, this means that we often feel hungry even when our bodies don't need more energy. If we eat anyways, we end up taking in more energy—or calories—than we need, so they get stored in our fat cells.

To a high degree, this frustrating cycle is caused by leptin or, more accurately, leptin dysregulation.

Leaning on Leptin

If you find yourself succumbing to hard-to-ignore cravings for food in the evening, even though you know you don't need any more energy, that is one very telling sign that you have an imbalance in your leptin levels.

One of the most interesting facts about this hormone is that it's released from fat cells, and therefore the amount of leptin produced by your body is directly related to the amount of body fat you have.

Leptin is your body's way of knowing how much body fat it has, which is an important biological safety net to keep you from starving during times of famine. When you have high leptin levels, your brain knows that you have adequate stores of body fat to keep you safe, theoretically setting systems in motion to allow you to eat less and burn more fat.

As your leptin levels decrease, your brain is signaled, and the systems reverse, causing you to eat more and burn less. Unfortunately, if the leptin receptors in your brain malfunction, your brain will continue to tell your body that it needs to consume and store more energy.

Leptin resistance is very similar to insulin resistance in that the more of this hormone that your body produces, the worse it's able to respond to it. The more energy you have stored in your fat cells, the more leptin is released, and the more resistant leptin receptors become.

Once again, we're faced with the reality that the problem is a hormonal imbalance that can't necessarily be addressed by the "eat less, exercise more" philosophy.

Consequences and Causes of Leptin Dysregulation

Anyone who has ever lost a considerable amount of weight because of a crash diet has probably also experienced the depressing effects of not only putting all the weight back on but actually even gaining more in the long-term.

You can thank leptin for this. When you lose a large amount of body fat in a short period of time, your leptin levels will drop dramatically, throwing your brain into a panic. The sudden lack of leptin signals danger and your brain will start screaming at you to eat more, and then it will take all the energy it can to refill the void in your fat cells.

Losing fat mass quickly on a calorically restrictive diet doesn't do anything to reverse leptin resistance, though, so even if you gain all the weight back, your hunger and storage signals won't turn off, causing you to pack on even more pounds.

If you lose weight by bringing your leptin hormones back into balance and healing leptin resistance, there won't be any reason for your brain to panic. Any weight loss will be gone for good, and as long as your leptin levels stay balanced, your weight will manage itself in the long-term.

The cause of leptin resistance is not 100% clear, but there are a few mechanisms that have been closely tied to the dysregulation of this particular hormone.

Chronically high leptin levels due to a high body fat index, as we've already discussed, is one clear culprit. Chronic inflammation also seems to be linked to the disorder, as well as having elevated levels of fatty acids in your bloodstream.

Balance Leptin Levels with Food

Everything about leptin acts as a one way street with two directions of traffic running through it.

Triglycerides are the most common type of fat in your body. Any energy that you consume and don't immediately burn for fuel is converted to triglycerides for storage. High triglyceride levels interfere with leptin transportation to your brain, throwing your hunger signals out of a healthy range.

If you can avoid putting on fat, leptin will help you avoid putting on fat.

Inflammation is another system that both increases leptin resistance and is exacerbated by having too much leptin in our bloodstream. If you can't control your levels of inflammation, leptin will help you control your levels of inflammation.

The confusing feedback system of leptin only occurs when it becomes dysregulated. Properly balanced leptin is a key figure in maintaining homeostasis in your body.

What to Eliminate and Avoid

Foods that are highly glycemic and can lead to weight gain will disrupt normal leptin production, so balancing your insulin in the previous reset will help significantly, but you'll want to continue consuming mostly low GI foods throughout this reset as well.

Avoiding inflammatory foods is the main focus of the next three days.

Processed foods, plants in the nightshade family, and FODMAPS will all be removed from your diet for the rest of the program.

Ideally, you'll already have nearly eliminated all processed foods by now, but if you haven't yet, it's high time you say goodbye to anything fried and fast. Processed foods contribute to unhealthy gut bacteria, destroyed microbiome, autoimmune disorders, and inflammation.

Nightshades contain a chemical called solanine, which, in some people, interfere with enzymes in your muscles, causing pain and stiffness. They can also increase inflammatory response, irritating your gut and joints. Whether or not you know you have a sensitivity to these foods, it's a good idea to avoid eating them to give your body a few weeks rest. Foods in the nightshade family include:

- potatoes, tomatoes, aubergines, and peppers

FODMAPs are fermentable carbohydrates that don't digest well. These carbs don't get absorbed into your bloodstream, but instead, travel all the way to the end of your gut, where the majority of your bacteria live. Once they're here, the bacteria begin to eat them, which can be great for a healthy microbiome, but in a damaged gut, it can create gas, increased digestive issues, and lead to inflammation.

To reduce FODMAPs in your diet, avoid the following:

- Fructose, found in primarily in low GI fruits, especially canned fruits

- Lactose, a carbohydrate from dairy products

- Fructans, present mainly in wheat products but also in smaller quantities in onions, garlic, and bananas

- Galatians, found in legumes and pulses

Some vegetables are also FODMAPs, containing any one of the above compounds. High FODMAP vegetables to avoid over the next three days include:

- Asparagus, Brussels sprouts, cauliflower, artichokes, leeks, and mushrooms

What to Enjoy More of

Reducing carbs and FODMAP foods can put a dent in the types of foods you're used to reaching for, but it provides a great opportunity for you to get experimental with your food choices.

Throughout the next three days, you'll want to increase your intake of soluble fiber, which supports gut health and protects against obesity. Increasing sources of high-quality protein will promote weight loss and help bring your leptin levels back to their optimal functioning levels.

High fiber, low FODMAP choices include:

- leafy greens like kale, spinach, arugula, swiss chard, collard greens, and lettuce

- sprouts, carrots, zucchini, cucumber, kohlrabi, radishes, and squashes

If you eat fruit, look for wild or organic and/or stick to berries. Modern fruit is genetically engineered to have more fructose than nature intended, not only making it more addicting but also making it harder to digest.

High protein, low FODMAP choices include:

- organic tofu, tempeh, and edamame
- pasture-raised organic eggs
- nuts and seeds

Additional Tips for Supporting Leptin

One of the most effective ways you can reset your leptin is to burn more fat. Of course, that's easier said than done.

You've probably heard that muscle burns more energy than fat does, which is why those with leaner body mass indexes tend to have faster metabolisms. While you can't alter your current body composition instantly, you can alter what you're giving your body to break down.

High protein meals are harder to break down than carbohydrates, which puts your metabolism to work. After eating a high protein meal, your metabolism can increase by as much as 30% for as long as 12 hours (Wellness Resources, 2008).

By starting your day with a high protein meal, instead of a high carb meal, you're setting your metabolism on overdrive for the entire day. Because it takes longer to break down, you will also feel full for a longer period of time, making it easier to make it through the 5 - 6 hours before your next meal without falling victim to cravings.

Improve Your Sleep

Leptin follows a circadian rhythm, which means that levels are at their highest in the evening. The most effective time your body has to make repairs is at night while you're sleeping. By establishing a consistent bedtime for yourself, your hormones will be better adapted to increase at the appropriate time, rather than being confused by sporadic sleeping patterns.

Leptin helps your body burn fat for fuel instead of glucose, so anything you can do to help it work effectively will improve your chances of losing weight naturally. Getting a good eight hours of sleep every night, especially if you're trying to lose weight, is a great way to support leptin regulation.

To improve your sleep and help your body spend more time repairing when you aren't sleeping, don't eat after dinner. Ideally, you'll want at least a 12-hour fasting window between your last meal of the day and your first meal of the next day.

Digestion is a very complex process that requires a lot of work. While your body is working hard on digesting your food, it doesn't have the resources needed to perform other functions, like repairing the damage done throughout the day.

If you eat your last meal 3 - 4 hours before you go to sleep, the vast majority of your digestive process will be complete, giving your body a full eight hours to do as much repair work as possible while you sleep.

Adapt to Intermittent Fasting

Giving your body a 12-hour window of fasting overnight is considered a low-intensity form of Intermittent Fasting (IF).

The longer you give your body to digest your food before giving it more work to do, the better your metabolic system is able to manage triglyceride levels better. Remember, a buildup of triglycerides can lead to leptin resistance.

Allowing enough time to fully digest your food before you eat again forces your body to start finding energy that is roaming through your bloodstream, not only preventing the excess energy from collecting in your fat cells but also helping your body more efficiently burn through excess fat that has already been stored. All in all, good digestion and fewer feedings per day helps you lose weight.

Constant grazing and snacking throughout the day can also affect insulin sensitivity, not only dysregulating multiple hormones but also causing you to eat more than you need to.

Instead of stressing yourself by counting every calorie you consume, simply try to avoid large meals and stop eating when you're not quite full.

We've talked about hormone cascades and how they take time to work through your bloodstream. For this reason, it can take 10 - 20 minutes for your hunger hormone, leptin, to completely turn off once you've ingested enough energy. If you eat until your 80 - 90% full, you'll more than likely find that after a short rest, you feel completely satiated. By eating your meal slowly, savoring each bite, you'll not only help your digestive system better process your food, but you'll also give your hormones more time to adjust your hunger signals properly.

Chapter 6:

Cortisol

Cortisol has a rather infamous reputation as the stress hormone. It's one of the hormones produced by your adrenal glands, and when it's running rampant through your bloodstream, this hormone can be the cause of significant damage.

But it's not just a villain.

Cortisol plays an important part in your overall health and safety as well, if it's properly balanced. We all need this hormone to help us cope in crisis situations, but it's important that we're able to effectively manage the hormone so that our body has time to relax and isn't always trying to put out fires.

The Good Side of Cortisol

There are four layers to your adrenal glands, each one producing a different hormone.

Epinephrine and norepinephrine, also known as adrenaline and noradrenaline, is responsible for the fight or flight response. It's controlled by your sympathetic nervous system (SNS) in a closely coordinated relationship with what is called the Hypothalamic-Pituitary-Adrenal Axis (HPA Axis).

The rest of the hormones produced by your adrenal glands are triggered through a hormone cascade that begins in the HPA Axis.

When you experience stress, your SNS activates adrenaline, which, in turn, speeds up your heart rate and begins to direct blood away from your digestive system and toward your muscles.

At the same time, a cascade of hormones trickle down from your hypothalamus to your pituitary gland, and finally to the adrenal cortices on top of your kidneys, triggering the release of cortisol.

Day to day, these hormones balance our blood sugar and blood pressure, but during a stress response, cortisol increases blood pressure, pumps glucose into your bloodstream, and shuts down non-emergency systems like digestion, immune response and reproductive development.

Once these stress hormones saturate your blood, eventually, your hypothalamus will get the message and want to reestablish homeostasis in your blood. It will stop producing the hormone that started the entire cascade, slowly but surely shutting down the stress response.

The Dangers of Excessive Cortisol

You've no doubt heard of the fight or flight response and how early humans needed this to survive from attacks of saber tooth tigers. As true as that may be, there aren't too many tiger related high-speed chases in the world today, but in 2006, a Canadian woman did wrestle a polar bear that was advancing on her son and his friend. She won that fight, thanks to a little help from the hormone partnership between adrenaline and cortisol (Waldie, 2018).

Unfortunately, if these super-human hormones stay elevated all day, every day, it can cause a number of problems.

The really tricky issue with cortisol is that it lingers in your blood until the hormones are broken down by enzymes, which can take some time. The longer cortisol stays in your bloodstream, the longer your digestive system, reproductive system, and immune response are turned off.

Because it dysregulates your digestive system, it can wreak havoc on your gut health and microbiome. Chronic high cortisol levels contribute to weight gain, specifically around your belly, where there is four times the number of cortisol receptors.

It should help you feel more alert to your immediate surroundings, but it shuts off brain function related to memory and has been linked to Alzheimer's disease and other permanent cognitive issues. It's been known to accelerate the aging process in other ways as well, contributing to muscle loss, a decrease in collagen, and even osteoporosis.

Another hormone that we're going to look at more closely in a few chapters is the growth hormone. The growth hormone helps to balance cortisol. The more growth hormone, the less cortisol, and vice versa. Unfortunately, as we age, we start to produce less growth hormone, and cortisol levels are thrown even further out of balance.

Balance Cortisol Levels with Food

Since a huge majority of people are suffering from an extreme excess of this particular hormone, for the rest of this reset, your goal is to reduce cortisol as much as humanly possible.

There are many lifestyle factors that relate to cortisol production, but taking stimulants to help you keep up with the stress of daily life can actually compound the damage stress itself does to your body.

What to Eliminate and Avoid

The two most common stimulants used in the 21st century are caffeine and sugar. Since we've already addressed sugar in resetting your insulin, it's time to talk about coffee.

Caffeine, which actually includes teas, energy drinks, soda, and even chocolate, can be a really effective stimulant when used in moderation. If over-consumed, it can overstimulate your nervous system, leading to exhaustion. This can result in anxiety, heart palpitations, and disrupted sleep.

Two factors that you'll see recurring often in

relation to your overall health is stress reduction and high-quality sleep. Caffeine sabotages both of them.

The health effects of coffee have been debated for generations, with no clear winning side. Some experts tell you to drink as much as possible because it's the largest source of antioxidants for most Americans.

Others will tell you that it can lead to cancer.

If you're following the recommendations of this reset, you'll be eating plenty of richly colored vegetables, so you shouldn't need coffee to serve as your antioxidant solution. And if you can get your hormones under control again, you should have to be concerned about coffee giving you cancer either.

But for at least the next three days, and preferably until the end of this reset, you will learn how to survive without artificial stimulation. The truth is, you shouldn't need stimulation to stay energized throughout the day, that is what calories, combined with quality sleep, are for.

Artificial stimulation of your hormones confuses the normal process of communication within your body, and our goal throughout this program is to put everything back into balance.

Aside from caffeine, the only other thing you'll be encouraged to eliminate entirely is stress eating. When you're stressed out, you more likely to reach for comfort foods that negatively affect how your body produces hormones in the long term.

Before you eat outside of your normal meal times, curb your stress eating tendencies by practicing some of the stress reduction techniques outlined throughout this book.

What to Enjoy More of

Part of the addiction to caffeine is the simple process of drinking. Replacing your regular coffee, tea, or soda with something else may not give you the caffeine hit you're used to, but it can help you feel like you're still filling the void.

If you're prone to ordering creamy, sweet lattes, you might want to try a "Golden Milk." This drink is gaining in popularity and is even available in many coffee chains. Starting with warmed organic, pasture-raised cow's milk or unsweetened plant-based milk alternatives, turmeric and other spices, such as cinnamon or ginger, are added.

If antioxidants are your goal, you cannot go wrong with this powerhouse. Turmeric is well known to help reduce inflammation, fight cell damage, boost brain power, protect against heart disease, improve symptoms of mood disorders, regulate blood glucose, and even defend you against cancer.

If black coffee is more your speed, there are mushroom elixirs that have an earthy flavor and color that will attract you. Specialty mushrooms have equally specialized antioxidants that help you focus, improve immune function, and even encourage relaxation.

If you primarily drink black tea, try switching to herbal teas. There are many flavors to choose from, so it can be a fun adventure to find one or more that you love. Just beware of sleepy time tea while you're at work.

Finally, if you crack open sodas or energy drinks regularly, try naturally flavored carbonated waters or kombucha, a fermented tea drink that is an incredible probiotic, which will enhance your gut microbiome. Just be sure to look for varietals made from herbal teas, as anything made from black tea or green tea will still have trace amounts of caffeine remaining.

Additional Tips for Lowering Cortisol Levels

Of course, when it comes to non-edible factors, it's important to stress once again just how big of factor *stress* plays in a healthy balance of cortisol production. Taking away caffeine can be a significant stressor for many people, so you'll need to find ways to compensate.

Supplementation of key nutrients and minerals can be a big help, but so can further stress reduction techniques.

Supplements

Your goal should be to stimulate your metabolism, giving you the energy you need without stimulating your nervous system, making you jittery, and increasing your stress response.

Several studies suggest that B-vitamins can help inhibit cortisol and reduce symptoms of stress, particularly in women (Stachowitz & Lebiedzinska, 2016).

A high-quality B-complex supplement will give you a specially formulated combination of the potent vitamins, but you can also incorporate it naturally into your diet by using nutritional yeast.

Nutritional yeast has been used as a nutrient-dense flavoring agent for potentially thousands of years, but as a vegan diet has continued to rise in popularity, so has this unique fungus.

A single serving of nutritional yeast can provide up to 9g of protein as well as a significant portion of your recommended daily intake of Vitamins B-1, B-2, B-6, and B-12.

It has a somewhat nutty or cheesy flavor and is commonly used in dairy-free cheese alternatives.

Approximately 50% of Americans are deficient in magnesium, which happens to be a mineral that is involved in a cyclical relationship with cortisol (American Osteopathic Association, 2018).

Your body needs magnesium to respond to stress effectively, but cortisol depletes magnesium. To add to the problem, you need magnesium to absorb Vitamin D properly, which is another vitamin that has been shown to have positive effects on regulating cortisol.

Supplementing with magnesium, or at least eating plenty of magnesium-rich foods, is a great way to help balance cortisol. Green leafy vegetables, nuts, seeds, legumes, and cold water fish are good food sources.

Vitamin D is available in the supplement form as well, but it can also be soaked in through your skin with 15 -20 minutes of careful sun exposure each day.

Finally, a family of non-toxic plants called adaptogens can come to your rescue. These herbs have been used for centuries in ancient holistic healing techniques like Ayurveda and Chinese medicine, but they are resurging in popularity in popular culture. Though trendy does not always correspond to effective, in this case, it makes a very healthy selection of herbs more accessible to the public.

Adaptogens help your body adapt and deal with all varieties of stress.

Your body is designed to respond to muscle damage by making your muscles stronger. There is a growing body of evidence that suggests adaptogenic herbs can do the same thing, but for your adrenal glands. Instead of stress making you weaker and more vulnerable, your body will learn to respond more quickly and effectively with unavoidable exposure to stress.

Some supplements to look for include:

- ashwagandha, Holy Basil, licorice root, robiola, ginseng, and decaffeinated matcha

Stress Reduction Techniques

Oxytocin is sometimes called the "love hormone" because it's released when you're involved with social bonding. Hugging, laughter, and even cuddling your dog can release this hormone, which reduces the effect of stress.

Part of your challenge over the next three days, and hopefully for the rest of your life, is to schedule more time for social fun and enjoyment.

Getting your body moving is another great way to reduce cortisol levels, but you need to focus on calming, relaxing activities. Extreme exercise is actually going to increase cortisol further, whereas a leisurely walk out in nature for 20 - 30 minutes a day will do a lot more for your stress levels.

You might also want to try barre classes, Pilates, yoga, or an easy jog. The key is to find an activity that you enjoy doing that will help you relax. Encouraging friends to join you will maximize your stress reduction.

We talked about meditation and breathing techniques in <u>Chapter 2</u>, and if you haven't started practicing these yet, now is the time. Breathing exercises and meditation can help drastically reduce stress, lowering your cortisol levels significantly.

Some research has even shown that shallow breathing through your mouth while you can increase cortisol, so taking some time before bed to simply take in deep breaths through your nose can improve sleep quality and reduce stress.

Leptin and growth hormone regulation also require high-quality sleep, so relaxing before sleep helps on multiple levels.

Insulin-like growth factor (IGF-1) is very similar to growth hormone, but it's produced by your liver. It regulates fat burning and blood sugar levels when you're not eating–such as when you're sleeping.

Controlling your thoughts to avoid increasing stress before you fall asleep can be hard to do, as it's often a time when we start to reflect on the day we just finished and the one that is on its way. Practicing meditation can help stimulate a relaxed, peaceful, and healing mind to help you fall into a deep, restorative sleep.

Chapter 7:

Thyroid Hormones

Your thyroid is located in front of your trachea in your neck, and it's responsible for producing three key hormones: triiodothyronine (T3), thyroxine (T4), and calcitonin.

When we refer to thyroid hormones in the future, we're talking specifically about T3 and T4. Thyroxine, T4, is more prevalent in a hormone, but it's also weaker. T3 is about four times more potent, but a healthy, well-functioning endocrine system has the ability to convert T4 to T3, increasing effectiveness overall.

These hormones help regulate homeostasis in your body that, by now, you should understand your body's preferred condition. Maintaining optimal body temperature, skin moisture, blood pressure, digestive juices, and level of oxygen, calcium, and cholesterol in your blood are just a few of the tasks on your thyroid's to-do list.

We talked about the HPA Axis in relation to the production of cortisol, and a very similar system is responsible for the production of thyroid hormones, only now we're dealing with the Hypothalamic-Pituitary-Thyroid Axis (HPT Axis).

The cascade of hormones begins when homeostasis is thrown out of whack for one reason or another, and turn off again with negative feedback. Once there's too much thyroid hormone running through your blood– not being used–your hypothalamus and pituitary gland will sense it and stop stimulating the thyroid.

When you have a hormonal imbalance, your thyroid might not turn on and off appropriately.

Symptoms of Thyroid Dysfunction

Thyroid hormones that are doing their job properly will stimulate your appetite and digestion, enabling the breakdown of nutrients so they can be absorbed and put to work. Almost every cell in your body has receptors for thyroid hormones, so you can just imagine how vital these particular hormones are to your overall health.

There are two main types of thyroid conditions:

hyperthyroidism, which occurs when your thyroid produces too many hormones and hypothyroidism, which happens when it's not producing enough hormones.

Hypothyroidism typically causes slow metabolism, respiratory, and cardiovascular activity. This can translate to symptoms of fatigue, weight gain, hair loss, heavy menstrual cycles, constipation, and possibly feeling cold all the time.

A low functioning thyroid is thought to be caused primarily by either iodine deficiency or an autoimmune disorder called Hashimoto's thyroiditis.

Your thyroid cannot produce hormones without iodine. In fact, thyroid function is the only known use for iodine, but it's an important one.

A deficiency of this mineral will cause your thyroid to swell as your HPT Axis continues to direct trigger hormones to your thyroid, even though it can't keep up with the demand. The hormone cascade effective gets stalled, pooling excess trigger hormones into your thyroid, where they collect with nowhere to go. This can cause what is known as goiter and results in a sensitive, swollen lump in your neck.

On the opposite end of the spectrum, we find Hyperthyroidism or an overactive thyroid that produces too much thyroid hormones. This increases metabolism as well as respiratory and heart rates beyond safe levels. Unstable weight loss, insomnia, irritability, diarrhea, and heat intolerance are symptoms of an overactive thyroid.

Another autoimmune disorder, Graves' disease, is the most common cause of hyperthyroidism.

Autoimmune Disorders and Thyroid Hormones

Autoimmune diseases occur when the immune system starts to attack itself. When it's thyroid dysfunction in question, the body specifically destroys your thyroid, making it unable to respond to the need for thyroid hormones effectively.

In the case of hyperthyroidism, your immune system produces an antibody called thyroid-stimulating immunoglobulin (TSI), which mimics the trigger hormone produced by your pituitary gland in the HPT Axis cascade. Unfortunately, TSI does not turn off when there is enough thyroid hormone in your bloodstream, but it continues to trick your thyroid into thinking it needs to produce more hormones to maintain homeostasis.

There are prescriptions and surgeries that can help manage symptoms of autoimmune disorders and the resulting thyroid dysfunction, but these solutions won't heal your body. By addressing the root cause of the disorder, you can reset your thyroid hormones to function properly.

Before we move on, it's important that you understand that there's a difference between rebalancing your hormone levels in 72 hours and curing an autoimmune disorder. The foods you do or do not eat can certainly help start the process of healing your gut, but that kind of damage takes time to repair. This reset does ***not*** claim to heal or cure any diseases that you may be suffering from.

One of the areas that your thyroid hormone is very active is in your gastrointestinal (GI) tract. Thyroid hormone controls glandular secretions, specifically alkaline and intestinal fluid, that help the smooth muscle surrounding your GI tract move waste out of your body.

If you have too much T3 circulating, it can result in diarrhea. Too little, and you'll be constipated.

Both of these conditions can affect the bacteria that live in your gut.

When food doesn't break down and move out properly, it can create micro holes in your intestinal tract. Undigested food particles and proteins can sneak through these tears into your bloodstream, causing an autoimmune response. This is commonly known as "leaky gut syndrome."

In yet another disturbing cycle, dysregulated production of thyroid hormone can increase your chances of developing an autoimmune disorder, and autoimmune disorders are one of the primary culprits for dysregulating thyroid hormone.

Balance Thyroid Hormone with Food

In the US, hypothyroidism is more common than hyperthyroidism, which means that the balance is more commonly due to a lack of thyroid hormones. That being said, it's not uncommon to vacillate between the two conditions, similar to the highs and lows of blood glucose levels.

To help your body naturally reset to the appropriate balance of thyroid hormones, the thyroid itself needs to be supported. In other words, instead of trying to influence how much hormone is being produced, we want to support the gland itself so that it can better regulate its own production in the long term.

What to Eliminate and Avoid

You may have focused in on the need for iodine in thyroid function. Worldwide, iodine deficiency is the leading cause of hypothyroidism, but it's extremely rare in the US, so using your thyroid as an excuse to eat more salty snacks is not going to solve any problems. Paying attention to how much iodine you're ingesting is a good idea, though, because you don't want to confuse your thyroid by having too much.

Goitrogens are foods that block iodine absorption. Raw cruciferous vegetables and soy are the most common culprits. These vegetables can still be amazingly powerful for your overall health, and even balancing multiple hormones, but you'll want to steam them during the reset.

Beyond iodine regulation, there are certain food items that are known to be thyroid disruptors. In other words, they suppress thyroid function.

The first food item you're going to want to completely remove from your diet for the remainder of this reset is gluten. You may or may not have a sensitivity to gluten, but that isn't actually what is causing the problem in this case.

The proteins in gluten mimic the proteins that are in your thyroid. If you happen to have an autoimmune disease, which often remains undiagnosed, your immune response is going to be triggered every time you consume gluten.

Not only is this going to continue to damage your thyroid, but it will also trigger an immune reaction throughout your body, worsening symptoms of inflammation, fatigue, and more.

Refined and processed grains, even those that are gluten-free, can cause similar immune responses due to similar proteins.

For best results, you want to stay far away from all of the following:

- bread, breakfast cereals, wheat, rye, barley, oats, millet, rice, spelled, etc.

Remember, you don't have to be gluten-free for the rest of your life, just long enough to reset your hormones and, if necessary, heal your gut.

Peanuts can also negatively disrupt your thyroid. They're not only goitrogens but also extremely acidic and inflammatory, and have been known to kill the good bacteria living in your gut. Your microbiome is crucial to a healthy immune response, so it's time to eliminate peanuts from your diet.

What to Enjoy More of

Eliminating gluten products from your diet can be a very difficult adjustment for most people who are used to the Standard American Diet (SAD). Before you go out in search of highly process gluten-free alternatives that are just going to add a lot of chemicals and toxins to your diet, consider sprouted grains and coconut flour products as a healthier alternative.

When grains are sprouted, their protein structure changes enough that your immune system shouldn't confuse them for thyroid hormones. The process of sprouting also kills off phytic acid, which allows your body to better absorb the nutrients from the grain, instead of storing them as fat (DoctorOz, 2014).

Next, if you're concerned that you can't even trade your favorite lunchtime sandwich in for peanut butter on celery, don't panic. You can still eat just about any other nut butter of your choice, but almond butter will have the most benefits. Almonds have a good supply of the amino acid L-arginine, which increases growth hormone, which we'll talk more about in the next chapter.

To support healthy gut bacteria, you'll want to get a good variety of fruits and vegetables that are high in fiber, which provide plenty of fuel for the good bugs in your stomach. Eating plenty of raw vegetables is great, but be sure to cook any cruciferous vegetables like broccoli and cauliflower.

For proteins, pasture-raised organic poultry and eggs are great for thyroid support, as is seafood. In fact, all high quality, organic pasture-fed meat can be healthy for those suffering from hypothyroid and gut health but wait until the end of the reset to add red meat back to your diet.

Probiotic foods are also incredible for your gut health. Some great choices can be:

- Fermented foods like kimchi, sauerkraut, pickled vegetables, tempeh, and miso
- Fermented beverages like kombucha, water, or coconut kefir

Once the 21-day reset is complete, you can also try adding in cultured dairy products like yogurt, buttermilk, and milk kefir. Some types of cheese are also probiotic, but look for labels that say "live" or "active cultures."

Raw nuts are also great for gut health, especially Brazil nuts. They're high in selenium, which is known to support your T3 and T4 production in your thyroid.

Additional Tips for Healthy Thyroid Function

Women are highly over-represented in statistics of thyroid dysfunction, being ten times more likely than men to develop hypothyroidism (Vanverpump, 2011).

Diet can have a major impact on your thyroid hormone production, but when you take into consideration what a close relationship it has with growth hormone and your sex hormones—estrogen, progesterone, and testosterone—it's a great idea to support this hormone in many ways as possible.

Understanding how your genetics factor into your thyroid health, as well as how you can influence those genetics in your favor, is important, as is avoiding as many environmental toxins and stressors that might have a negative impact on your genetics is also an effective way to be proactive about your future health.

Genetics and Epigenetics

Many health disorders seem to run in the family, and that's often because of our genetics. Thyroid disorders are one of these potentially hereditary health disorders. But blaming unbalanced thyroid hormones entirely on your genetics is not only an incomplete truth, but it's also defeatist and unhelpful.

While you may have a genetic predisposition to poor thyroid health, your DNA doesn't have to have the final say.

Epigenetics can also help you determine and self-regulate your own fate.

Your genes can exist in your body in either an activated state or a deactivated state. If a gene is deactivated, it won't cause the disruption that it's potentially capable of.

Factors outside your genetics influence whether or not your genes get turned on. Even if every woman in your family has been diagnosed with thyroid disorders, there is still hope that your own personal disorderly genes will never get turned on.

What kind of factors influences your epigenetics? Diet, exposure to chemicals and environmental toxins and stressors, physical fitness, social experiences, trauma, and some medications.

If you find this hard to believe or accept, think about identical twins. They have the exact same DNA and genetics, but over time, they become more and more individualized as they each interact differently with their environment, activating or deactivating certain genes in different ways.

A positive note in relation to epigenetics is that once a gene is turned on—or off for that matter—it doesn't necessarily have to stay that way.

A healthy diet, regular physical activity, and low exposure to contaminants can help your epigenetics return to their optimal health-inducing state.

Environmental Toxins and Stressors

With your genetics in mind, there are a few specific environmental toxins and stressors that have been known to influence how your thyroid hormones get expressed.

First of all, severe carb restriction can increase reverse T_3 production, which blocks thyroid receptors.

T_3 is the active form of thyroid hormone that boosts your metabolism and stimulates the use of fat in your cells for energy. Reverse T_3 is the inactive form, which doesn't just mean that it's "off," it also works against your metabolism, stopping your fat-burning potential.

Because your thyroid requires iodine, which is a halogen, as well as selenium, which is a metalloid, to function properly, it is particularly susceptible to damage from similar, yet harmful, halogens and heavy metals. Industrial chemicals, herbicides and pesticides, toxins in beauty products and other household commodities, and heavy metals can severely damage your thyroid.

We'll talk more about how to mitigate the effects of environmental toxins in Chapter 9.

Finally, your thyroid is also sensitive to disruptions in your other hormones, such as estrogen and testosterone, leptin, growth hormone, and cortisol. If you're one of the many women suffering from a thyroid disorder, committing to this reset will help from multiple angles.

Chapter 8:

Growth Hormone

The growth hormone is linked very closely to the aging process. Starting in your 30s, your body starts to produce less growth hormone naturally.

Among other responsibilities, growth hormone helps to balance cortisol. The more growth hormone your body produces, the lower your cortisol levels will be. As you produce less growth hormone, you not only have to deal with the immediate results of this deficiency, but you also have to cope with even more dysregulated cortisol.

How Growth Hormone Works

The growth hormone is produced directly in your pituitary gland, triggered by stimulating hormones produced by your hypothalamus.

There are five main factors that stimulate the production of GH:

1. high amino acid levels in the blood
2. low blood glucose/hypoglycemia
3. low fatty acids in the blood
4. healthy stressors
5. exercise

Once stimulated, the growth hormone goes to work, trying to balance out the first three stimulating factors with a goal of lowering amino acid levels in your blood and increasing blood glucose and fatty acid levels.

Some of the hormones will bind with target receptors on your liver and eventually gets converted to Insulin-like Growth Factor 1 (IGF-1).

IGF-1 promotes protein synthesis by binding with receptors on your skeletal muscle cells, encouraging the absorption of amino acids, balancing out the first stimulating factor.

When amino acids link together, they create proteins. Since this is specifically happening inside your muscle cells, the new amino acid chains increase the size of the muscle and improve function.

When the growth hormone interacts with your liver, it stimulates the process of gluconeogenesis. Remember, it was called as a response to low blood glucose levels, so now it wants to rebalance them. The hormone binds to receptors on adipose tissue, activating an enzyme called hormone-sensitive lipase. This starts to break down triglycerides that are stored in your fat cells into glycerol and fatty acids.

This process effectively raises blood glucose and fatty acid levels while it burns fat. Adequate levels of growth hormone can really come to your aid when you're trying to lose weight.

When IGF-1 interacts with your bones, it increases bone deposition and resorption, helping your bones grow thicker and stronger. It also works inside your cartilage, encouraging interstitial growth, or lengthening.

As you age and produce less growth hormone, your bones can become more brittle, and your cartilage depletes, reducing mobility and stability of your bones.

Signs and Causes of Growth Hormone Imbalance

The Hormone Reset Diet is primarily concerned with balance. You don't want too much or too little of any hormone, and you want your body's natural functioning to be able to discern and produce exactly the right amount when, and only when it's needed.

Low growth hormone production can lead to mood changes like anxiety, minor depression, and general feelings of unease. If you're not producing enough growth hormone, you'll likely feel fatigued and probably have issues with weight gain.

Many of the so-called "normal" signs of aging are also symptoms of low growth hormone.

Growth hormone deficiency is more commonly diagnosed in children when they, quite noticeably, stop growing at the expected rate. It frequently happens in adults, as well. However, the symptoms are often ascribed to various other potential causes.

It's often triggered by damage to the pituitary gland, hypothalamus, or the receptors involved in regulated growth hormone.

Balance Growth Hormone with Food

We haven't yet talked about pH balance in your body, but it's another very important predictor of overall health.

Your neural, or balanced, pH is 7. Anything less than that is considered alkaline, and if it is higher than that, it's acidic.

The Standard American Diet (SAD) sabotages pH levels. Coffee, dairy, animal products, sugar, simple carbs, and fried foods all tilt the scale toward acidity and are consumed regularly by Americans. On the other hand, leafy greens and vegetables, which are consumed in my lower proportion, the trend toward alkaline.

The growth hormone is influenced by pH levels in your blood, being suppressed when you're acidic, and flourishing in an alkaline environment (Schwalfenberg, 2011).

As we discussed in the previous chapter, thyroid hormone is critical in the production of growth hormone, so anything that disrupts your thyroid function, particularly food intolerances and autoimmune disorders, will also affect your growth hormone production.

What to Eliminate and Avoid

Gluten has been the most inflammatory item removed from your diet so far, but for the next three days specifically, and preferably for the remainder of the reset, you're going to remove dairy.

The vast majority of food intolerances come from one of these two substances, and removing them from your diet for a short period of time will help your gut heal, whether or not you are personally sensitive to them.

Dairy is well known to be a significant cause of inflammation in your body. A healthy immune system responds to injury and sickness by protecting the damaged area with inflammation. Unfortunately, chronic inflammation is thought to be the root cause of almost all preventable diseases and is most certainly a contributing factor to weight gain and resistance to weight loss.

By removing dairy from your eating plan, you're highly likely to notice a reduction in symptoms like fatigue, IBS, anxiety, and fluid retention or bloating.

Approximately 75% of people around the world have difficulty processing lactose, the carbohydrate found in dairy. Percentages increase for those of African American, Asian, Native American, or Mexican American descent, and also for anyone with gluten sensitivity.

As you age, your body stops being able to produce the enzyme lactase, which is needed to break down the lactose in dairy. This results in highly uncomfortable digestive distress, leading to bloating and gas, diarrhea, and/or gastroesophageal reflux (GERD), which you'll feel in the form of heartburn.

Dairy is a major trigger for dysregulated gut health, specifically the proteins casein and whey.

Casein is a protein in milk that your immune system frequently mistakes for an intruder, creating an aggressive immune response against it, usually representing like allergies: skin reactions, sneezing, itchy eyes, possible swelling of lips, tongue, mouth or throat and, in severe cases, anaphylaxis

Whey is a different protein that will cause a similar, though unrelated, immune response. Whey can be harder to avoid because it's commonly used in protein supplements and food products, so read labels carefully!

Women have a more sensitive immune response than men, which is great in a healthy body, but if your microbiome is damaged or your hormones are unbalanced, it puts you at a much higher chance of developing an autoimmune disorder.

What to Enjoy More of

By removing dairy from your diet, you'll also be removing key nutrients that are either naturally occurring in milk products or added to them. As such, you'll want to focus on integrating high-quality alternative sources of calcium, potassium, and vitamin D.

For calcium, you can increase your intake of:

- chia seeds are a great source of dairy-free calcium because they're also high in boron, which helps your body actually to metabolize the calcium effectively

- almonds, sunflower seeds, and sesame seeds have high levels of calcium as well as healthy fats

- tofu, white beans, and edamame are not only excellent sources of dairy-free calcium, but they're all high in clean protein as well

- for vegetables, consider adding broccoli rabe, kale, sweet potato, collard greens, arugula, and butternut squash to your menu

Most fruits and vegetables are rich in potassium, so as long as your eating plenty of plant-based foods, you shouldn't need to worry about this mineral.

Dairy-free sources of Vitamin D:

- most milk alternatives will be fortified with vitamin D, just like dairy is, so make the simple swap to organic soy, almond, coconut, or hemp milk

- Fish, particularly salmon, mackerel and trout are also high in Vitamin D

- Egg yolks are also great sources of vitamin D, just make sure you are opting for pasture-raised, organic eggs for quality

Additional Tips for Naturally Regulating Growth Hormone

Removing dairy from your eating plan might be a bit of a painful process, but the more you know about what you're eating, the more determined you'll be to clean up your dietary habits.

To help stimulate healthy production of growth hormone, you can also subject your body to some healthy stressors as opposed to the negative, damaging stress that causes dysregulation.

How you move your body and how often you exercise can have a big impact on the proper regulation of growth hormone in your body. If you want to tap into this "fountain of youth," you'll have to pay just as much attention to your exercise routine as your eating patterns.

Exercise

One of the most effective ways to increase growth hormone through physical exercise is to practice High-Intensity Interval Training (HIIT) or burst exercise a few times a week.

Generally, it involves sprinting of sorts. For a short burst, usually around 20 - 30 seconds, you push your body to about 80% of your maximum heart rate, and when you return to a few minutes of low-intensity movement. You would repeat this 4 - 5 times over a 20 -30 minutes exercise session.

By incorporating high-intensity bursts, you increase your VO2 max, which is the amount of oxygen you're consuming.

In regular aerobic exercise, your body will take in more oxygen to fuel the workout. Oxygen alone isn't enough to support the anaerobic bursts involved in HIIT, so your body starts to burn fat to keep up with the demand of your workout.

To do this, your body needs to increase the amount of growth hormone circulating in your blood.

Adding sprints to your exercise routine will also lower insulin levels by burning excess blood sugar.

Avoiding Conventional Animal Products

Hormones are regularly pumped into animals to fatten them up so that farms and farmers can make more money per animal. When you eat that meat, you're ingesting those hormones too… and they'll fatten you up as well.

This is especially true in the dairy industry, where the cows are injected with a variety of hormones that help them continue to produce great quantities of milk.

Anyone alive today is likely familiar with the saying, "does a body good," in reference to milk. It turns out this might be more of a marketing ploy than actual truth.

We've been raised to consider milk as a critical source of calcium, potassium, and vitamin D, believing it to be crucial to the development and maintenance of healthy bones.

There is actually very little reliable scientific backing for milk, and most of what's available can be associated with—in other words, paid for by the dairy industry, which makes it suspect at best. As we've already pointed out, there are plenty of non-dairy sources of healthy calcium that don't cause allergic reactions in 75% of people.

Dairy is also highly addictive. Casomorphins are opioids found in dairy that have powerfully addictive qualities. In a way, this is nature's foolproof method to make sure babies drink milk to grow.

But nature will eventually reduce milk supply, encouraging the weaning process. A healthy baby will only eat when hungry, so when solid foods start being introduced, they'll naturally drink less breast milk, gradually weaning them off without causing severe symptoms of withdrawal.

When adults consume dairy regularly, and in high quantities, they become addicted.

Moreover, the hormones in milk concentrate in fat, which is why many people have a harder time giving up cheese, which has a high-fat content than skim milk, for example.

You may experience withdrawal symptoms when you eliminate dairy, but once you've broken your addiction, it will lose much of its appeal, making it easier to say "no" to dairy the longer you abstain from it.

Chapter 9:

Testosterone

Just as women naturally produce more estrogen hormones, men naturally produce more testosterone hormones. Testosterone boosts metabolism and helps the owners of said hormone stay lean, more easily burning fat and building muscle mass. In a world where excess weight is not overly desirable, this may strike a lot of women as "unfair."

Similar to progesterone production, as women age–especially after 35–testosterone production decreases steadily. Testosterone production goes down with each of these conditions:

- Post-menopause

- ovary removal or decrease of ovarian function caused by chemotherapy

- Pituitary or adrenal gland dysfunction

In men, the production of testosterone is one of the primary concerns of the testes. Women obviously don't have testes, but the small amount of testosterone they do produce is divided between their ovaries and adrenal glands.

Many of the suggestions made in the first reset that encouraged the lowering of estrogen will have a similar balancing effect on testosterone. You've been working on this hormone right from the start!

Testosterone Effects

Testosterone is a sex hormone, so its primary purpose is dedicated to increasing reproductive and sexual function. Having too much or too little of this hormone can result in a loss of libido, but having too little can also cause fertility issues.

The hormone is also designed to help your body build muscle and burn body fat, as well as enhance mood. Imbalances in this hormone, even though women require very little of it, can have significant side effects.

Low testosterone is more common because it has an inverse relationship to estrogen. When estrogen is high, testosterone dips low and vice versa. Some consequences of low testosterone include:

- increase in signs of aging, such as wrinkles, rapid muscle loss, which is undesirable on its own, but also leads to saggy skin and bone density issues like osteopenia or osteoporosis

- symptoms of menopause, such as hot flashes, irritability, mood swings, and reproductive challenges

- low sex drive, weakness, fatigue, thinning hair

In extreme cases, low testosterone has even been linked to cardiovascular disease and cancer.

High testosterone, on the other hand, is less common but has equally severe consequences.

- an increase in masculine traits, such as abnormal body hair growth, male pattern baldness, deepening voice, shrinking breasts, and irregular menstrual cycles

- increased body fat, especially around the midsection

A little goes a long when it comes to testosterone in a woman's body, and an imbalance can be dangerous.

Causes of Unbalanced Testosterone

Endocrine disruptors, particularly found in birth control and environmental toxins, are confusing our body's natural communication system, making it nearly impossible to *naturally* produce the correct amount of sex hormone for optimal health.

Damage or disruption to glands that produce complementary hormones, such as your adrenals, thyroid, and pituitary, can also cause an imbalance of your testosterone production, either high or low, depending on the relationship with the triggering hormones.

Low testosterone in women is becoming endemic, at least in part due to the prevalence of other imbalanced hormones, particularly estrogen.

Raised levels of cortisol, as you know, cause you to gain and store fat, especially around the midsection. It also contributes to poor sleep quality and dysregulated blood sugar. The cortisol spike itself, as well as the results of high cortisol, all act against the natural production of testosterone.

Low-fat diets, as well as statin drugs that are made to lower cholesterol, can also cause low testosterone.

High testosterone in women is most commonly caused by taking exogenous testosterone supplements, adrenal disorders, and a condition called PCOS, or polycystic ovarian syndrome.

PCOS doesn't currently have a definitive known cause, but it is thought to be related to metabolic disorders and high insulin.

Balance Testosterone with Food

It's clear that the human body is designed to cope with stress and toxins, but not at the level we're currently exposing ourselves to. When it comes to balancing your testosterone levels with food, it is more important that you pay attention to the production and storage than the food itself.

We're exposed to hundreds, if not thousands of toxins every day, from the cosmetics and beauty products we put on our skin and hair, to the cleaners and household items we handle. Even the air we breathe and the water we drink contain toxins and heavy metals that can damage our endocrine system.

While we can't eliminate them all, we can try not to ingest them on purpose.

Unless it's certified organic, environmental toxins in our food include:

- pesticides and herbicides
- fertilizers
- synthetic hormones

Looking at the materials, your food is packaged and stored in is also important, as aluminum cans and plastic are known to be very damaging to your health.

What to Eliminate and Avoid

Endocrine disruptors, and particularly estrogen disruptors, are found in the chemicals that are used to grow your food and the plastics you store your food in. In order to avoid adding more to the already overwhelmed state of your body, you'll have to change a few shopping habits.

You've probably heard of BPA, or bisphenol A. It's a chemical used to make plastics and resins and rose in infamy over the past few years for being associated with infertility and a host of other health disorders.

You may or may not be familiar with the consequences, but you've no doubt seen plenty of products claiming to be "BPA free." This alone creates the impression that you want to avoid it. The problem is that, while BPA might be on everyone's radar, BPF and BPS and other BPA substitutes that have nearly the same chemical makeup are being used instead.

Calling attention to one toxin to hide the presence of another is a very effective marketing technique. Just because you choose water bottles and Tupperware containers that are BPA free does not mean they are safe for your health (Gregor, M., 2017).

When you store your food or buy packaged food items, which are hopefully becoming less common on your grocery lists, prioritize glass or stainless steel containers that won't leach harmful chemicals in your food.

Liquids can be particularly susceptible, so be highly conscious of your beverage choices.

If you must use plastic containers, keep them away from heat at all times. Don't heat up your food in plastic, put food into plastic containers while it's still hot, or even leave it exposed to sunlight. Plastic has been shown to leach chemicals out of plastic and into your food by 55 faster when it's heated (Biello, 2008).

What to Enjoy More of

First and foremost, you want to do everything you can to support your liver, your body's primary detoxifying organ. Choosing foods based on specific minerals and nutrients is a good start, but you also want to make sure you aren't adding more toxins to your body in the process.

Now more than ever, it's important that you buy organic produce whenever possible. The chemicals and pesticides used on conventional crops are highly disruptive to your body's natural production of estrogen, which, in turn, dysregulates testosterone production.

Some of the most beneficial minerals for your liver are:

- Magnesium, best consumed in leafy greens, nuts and seeds, legumes, and cold-water fish such as salmon, mackerel and tuna

- Sulfur, which can be found in coconut and olive oils, radishes, watercress, arugula, kale, broccoli, Brussels sprouts, blue-green algae, spirulina, hemp, pumpkin seeds

- Selenium has the highest concentration in Brazil nuts

- Zinc and Copper are often found in the same foods, particularly in shellfish like oysters and lobster, an alga called spirulina, nuts, seeds, and legumes

One further food item that you might want to consider to support your liver is, in fact, liver. It is considered a superfood by many because it's packed with healthy protein, vitamins, and minerals are crucial to your survival.

If you enjoy the liver, make sure you are eating a healthy liver. Always choose organic, hormone-free, pasture-raised organ meat and ethics allowing, the younger liver, the better, so calf or lamb liver can be especially potent.

Bone broth is also a helpful way to help your liver remove toxins from your body, and it helps in the repair process as well. There are amino acids in bone broth that stimulate collagen production, encouraging a healthy inflammation response in your body as well as tightening and toning your skin.

Finally, you want to make sure you're drinking plenty of clean, filtered water. This is not the same as bottled water, which not only comes in plastic, but it often is no different than the water from your tap. Getting a simple, activated carbon or charcoal water filter for your fridge at home is an inexpensive way to help you drink more healthy, clean water to support your body's natural detoxification process.

Additional Tips for Supporting Testosterone Levels

Testosterone production is one of your hormones that is heavily influenced by the environment you are situated in, every day. Yes, of course, stress is a large factor, but how you move your body and what types and varieties of external toxins you're exposed to play a critical role as well.

Sex hormones are one of the easiest for medical science to synthetically duplicate, which is why women are often prescribed birth control to deal with excess estrogen-related issues. Synthetic testosterone is also frequently prescribed, as is medication designed to block testosterone receptors, depending on whether your body is producing too much or too little of the hormone.

But just because we *can* trick our body into thinking everything is rebalanced, doesn't mean we necessarily *should*.

Exercise

Naturally stimulating your endocrine system to produce, use, and eliminate testosterone as your body actually requires is the best solution to hormone management. One of the simplest ways to do this is to exercise.

Yoga helps to realign your entire body, inside and out, improving digestion and natural detoxification. It also improves breathing, and oxygen is a powerful natural detoxification tool.

Resistance or weight training to build muscle stimulates growth hormone and testosterone production. A lot of women get nervous at the idea of weight training because they don't want to end up looking bulky and masculine. This is not a very substantial risk, however, because even men have to work really hard to get bulky themselves, and they naturally produce a lot more testosterone. It's rare for women to get bulky and only happens with specific training measures and supplementation.

Balancing your hormones isn't about producing a lot of testosterone; it's about producing the right amount of testosterone for health.

Interval training, using sprints, bursts, or HIIT has also been shown to increase the production of both growth hormone and testosterone, and as an added bonus, this method of training is the least time consuming to see results.

Supplements vs. Medications

There are plenty of frequently prescribed medications and bioidentical hormones that can synthetically "balance" your hormones. What they really do is drive your levels beyond their normal range, regardless of how your biological system responds to them. In other words, there is no "off" button to medications.

There are a place and time for everything, but if you're using medicine or bioidentical hormones, you have to monitor all your hormone levels carefully and often. They may also have a negative effect on HDL, so it's a good idea to monitor cholesterol as well.

Generalizing the situation, medications suppress and hide symptoms, whereas holistic measures help address the root cause to heal the problem.

Diet and lifestyle changes aren't introducing hormones to your body; they're stimulating the natural production of hormones for optimal, balanced biological processes to occur.

In addition to the changes already encouraged, you can also look into a family of herbs called "adaptogens." These are plants that help your body adapt to and deal with stressors. They were mentioned briefly in Chapter 6 as a way to manage cortisol levels, and that practice can also help balance your testosterone.

Ashwagandha, for example, has been shown to decrease cortisol, increase DHEA, and thereby increase free testosterone levels. Look for a root extract that includes 'withanolides."

Toxins and Heavy Metals

Understanding the dangers of toxins and heavy metals are important, but it might also help to understand how they are stored and released into your body.

All hormones interact with cells using receptors that are either inside the cell, for fat-soluble hormones, or along the outer cell wall, in the case of water-soluble hormones.

Toxins and heavy metals are often stored in adipose or fat tissues and are difficult to get rid of because your body is protecting itself from the toxins by hiding them away in your fat cells where they can't do much damage.

Sex hormones are all fat-soluble, so while these toxins are hiding out in your fat cells, they disrupt your hormone receptors for estrogen, progesterone, testosterone, cortisol, and thyroid hormone. You may have noticed that these hormones interact very closely with each other.

Metals that are known to accumulate in your body include:

- mercury, cadmium, lead, and arsenic

Some level of heavy metals is expected, and your body can handle. Unfortunately, overexposure has made toxicity a problem.

There are many ways humans are exposed to heavy metals and other endocrine-disrupting chemicals, such as:

- passed on through pregnancy/birth
- environmental factors: toys, paint, household items
- work: construction industry, salons, printing industry
- dental work: metals and/or mercury in fillings
- antiperspirants and aluminum foil
- vaccines: particularly in the past, mercury compounds were used in vaccines as a preservative

- processed foods and natural foods: these metals are in the soil, which means they're in the plants and everything that eats plants

- cosmetics and hygiene products: especially look out for parabens, phthalates, sodium lauryl sulfate, each of which is well-known estrogen-mimicking chemicals
- Toxicity has been linked to serious diseases and disorders:

- autism, ADD, ADHD are linked to heavy metal toxicity

- cancer

- imbalanced immune system

- syndromes such as IBS and fibromyalgia

- neurodegenerative diseases like Alzheimer's, Parkinson's and Dementia

Everything you're doing to heal your natural testosterone balance can also help remove toxins from your body. When you detox a lot of toxins rapidly, as happens when you lose a lot of weight quickly or suddenly integrate detoxing agents into your eating plan, you might not be able to eliminate them quickly enough, and your body will start to reabsorb them, fitting them back into your fat cells.

If this happens on mass, you may experience symptoms like gas, bloating, skin rash, loose bowels, or nausea. In other words, you may feel worse before you feel better.

Chapter 10:

What to do after Your Reset

The last thing you want to do after going through the commitment of the past 21 days is to return to old habits that will throw your hormones right back out of sync. You don't have to be on a diet for the rest of your life, but you should establish new patterns of eating that will support your hormones and your overall health.

Now that your hormones are back in balance, it'll be much easier to understand the cues your body is giving you. Without the confusion and mixed messages of a broken metabolism, your body should be telling you the truth more often than not now.

It's your job to learn to listen to your body and understand what it's telling you, instead of selectively intuiting only what you want to hear. When you give your body a chance to heal, you might be surprised at how often you crave "healthy" foods instead of items that never fail to make you feel guilty.

Gradually Reintegrate Food

As you finalize your hormone reset, you can start to reintroduce eliminated foods back into your meal planning.

Try not to rush this process, but do so gradually by consuming them one at a time, once per day, for at least a couple of days before moving onto another reintroduction. By adding foods back one at a time, you'll not only give your gut time to readapt to the food, but you'll also know instantly if that food causes any problems for you. Your metabolism and digestive system will react instantly to any irritants, and it will be obvious what is causing the sensitivity.

Listen to your gut. If bloating, heartburn, or either constipation or diarrhea are a reaction to a change in your eating habits, don't ignore these signs. It's far better to live healthfully for the rest of your life without a particular food than to damage your body and live in pain and discomfort for the rest of your life.

Practice Mindful Eating

Before you reintroduce something that you haven't had in the past 21 days, ask yourself why you're adding it back into your eating plan. Is it to work your way back to a healthy, balanced, and sustainable eating plan? If yes, go for it, but start with small portion sizes to let your body adjust, and take notes about how your body reacts.

If you're reintroducing something that instantly makes you feel guilty, reconsider. You've just treated your body like a goddess for 21 days, do you really want to slide back into bad habits? You've come this far, if you don't want to have to detox and go through withdrawal again in six months, maybe you should just keep certain destructive foods out of your life for good. It will never be easier than now when you're healthier than you've probably been in years, and you've already kicked symptoms of withdrawal.

Practicing mindful eating can help you listen to your body's signals. Start paying close attention to *why* you're eating, whether you're actually hungry, or if you're trying to fill some other need. If you're eating for a non-hunger related issue, find something else to fill that void.

If you think you're hungry, but it's not a proper mealtime, drink a glass of water and spend five minutes doing something else to occupy your mind. If you're still hungry, have a healthy snack, like a handful of nuts. If your hunger is gone, or if you forget that you were hungry, don't eat!

If you have a craving for something specific that isn't on your ", feel great" foods list, reference the swaps list you created at the beginning of a plan. If you're hungry for something sweet, but a banana doesn't appeal to you, you're probably not hungry. Maybe you're bored, emotional, or procrastinating, and there's a better way to handle the issue.

Do you remember the days before the hormone reset when you would grab yourself a snack at night and then sit down in front of the television to enjoy your favorite show? We've all done that. No matter how determined you are to just have a few bites of this ice cream or only a handful of those chips, half an hour goes by, and we look down to find the entire pint demolished or bag emptied. Not only did you just consume a load of empty calories, but you weren't even really present enough to enjoy them!

Mindful eating is about focusing on each bite, savoring and appreciating the food you're eating, and removing distractions that lead to overeating and binge eating.

Think about actually chewing your food while you eat. The more you chew, the better you'll digest it. Also, the more in tune you are with the process of eating, the less likely you are to overeat accidentally.

Mindful eating can help you better appreciate, taste, and cherish your food.

Intermittent Fasting (IF)

Each of the hormonal imbalances we addressed over the past 21 days, particularly insulin, leptin, and cortisol, influence and are influenced by your appetite and eating patterns.

Intermittent fasting allows you to adequately rest your body, allowing it the time it needs to heal. By depleting your reserves of energy, you'll reset your entire body to function more like it did before weight was ever a problem for you.

IF has been proven to help fat burning and sustained weight loss without restricting or even counting calories.

Adjust For Sensitivities and Intolerances

As mentioned a few times already in this chapter, it's important for your long-term health that you adjust your eating plan moving forward to completely eliminate any foods that might trigger a hormonal or autoimmune response.

Having eliminated many common sensitivities for days, if not weeks, puts you in a perfect situation to notice exactly what might be bothering you, without wondering which of the ten items you ate for dinner triggered your heartburn today.

This is a good point to enlist the help of your doctor or a nutritionist, registered dietician or naturopathic professional, if you haven't already. They can perform simple sensitivity tests that should provide you with clear results now that your body has done some healing and is thinking more clearly.

Moving forward, your focus when you eat should always be to integrate as many clean, nutrient-dense foods as possible and eliminate as many empty calories and chemical/additive-laden foods as you can.

Eliminate for life:

There are some foods, beverages, and food-like items that should simply never have a place on your plate.

Conventionally produced meat and dairy are loaded with hormones and antibiotics which destroy your hormone balance and the gut microbiome.

In 2014, more than 20 million pounds of antibiotics were sold for use in animal agriculture, which represents around 80% of the total antibiotics sold during that year (Foodprint.org, 2019).

Antibiotics have saved millions of lives, and they are an incredible advancement of modern medicine, but there is no denying the fact that they also interfere with gut health and hormone balance.

If you are prescribed antibiotics to heal from a disease or injury, they might be critical to your survival. However, if you're eating them without even knowing they're in your food, they are damaging your long-term health, rather than helping it. 80% of antibiotics being pumped into conventionally farmed meat puts your health at risk.

That doesn't even take into consideration the steroid hormones being injected into livestock to make them grow big and fatty. Those hormones will also make you grow big and fatty.

Even without antibiotics and hormones to consider, industrially produced animal agriculture is typically grain-fed. These animals are lower in nutrition because they're not getting the natural vitamins (A, B, C & E) or fatty acids (omega 3s) that grass-fed animals ingest normally.

Moving forward, conventionally produced meat and dairy should not be on your grocery list, and neither should any processed meats that are filled with preservatives and additives.

There are also some oils and fats that you're going to want to avoid permanently. Healthy, natural fats are great for your body and metabolism. Highly processed oils like vegetable oils—canola, soy, corn—and anything that says partially hydrogenated are not and should be avoided at all costs.

Finally, for your long-term health, look to the beverages that you're consuming. What you drink can be one of the quickest ways to influence your hormones, particularly insulin.

Stay far away from soda, commercial fruit juice, and energy drinks.

Some alcohol, coffee, and tea can be a good source of antioxidants, but their benefits are easily overcome by the detrimental burdens on your liver if you over-consume. Limit your intake, and try not to binge drink any of these beverages.

Finally, drink plenty of water, but keep it out of plastic bottles. Use stainless steel or glass bottles instead.

Enjoy for life

First, a little clarification. The last section was not meant to imply that you should never eat meat again. Instead, simply focus on organic, pasture-raised meat and dairy and eat it in moderation. Wild game can also be a tasty and healthy addition to your meal plan.

To supplement your meat, continue to eat cold-water fish that are low in mercury, like wild-caught salmon, cod, trout, sardines, anchovies. Shellfish also has many health benefits, so work crab, clams, oysters, and scallops into your cooking at least occasionally.

Finally, don't forget or forego your plant-based

proteins. Legumes, certain nuts and seeds, some whole grains, and organic soy products have dense nutritional profiles that will not only supplement your clean protein intake but also provide you with a healthy collection of additional vitamins and minerals.

Many of your healthiest fats will also be in your proteins, in the animal and seafood products you eat. Nuts, seeds, and avocados are fantastic plant-based sources of nutrient-dense, healthy fat, as are certain oils. Olive, avocado, and coconut oils are high in healthy mono and polyunsaturated fats, as is organic, pasture-raised ghee.

Fruits, especially berries, lemons, and limes, can be eaten in moderation for the rest of your life unless you have a sensitivity to them or some other metabolic disorder. They are high in nutrients and fiber and a great alternative to sweets, but they are still high in sugar, so eating too many fruits can disrupt insulin and other hormones again.

Vegetables can more or less exist in unlimited quantities in the future. As long as your unique and individual biological system doesn't have a sensitivity to a particular vegetable, eat them at will and in as much variety as you can manage.

Similarly, the sky's the limit in regard to plant-based herbs and spices. Go straight to the source and avoid packaged spice combinations that are extraordinarily high in salt and potentially have chemicals and other additives like MSG.

When you're thirsty, reach for filtered water first. Consider keeping cold, naturally flavored water in your fridge so that it's available whenever you need it. You can also slowly reintroduce tea and coffee in moderation, but drink them both without sugar or dairy if possible. Kefir and kombucha are healthy, probiotic drinks that will add plenty of variety to your life if you need something a little different.

With a well-balanced eating plan, you should get most of the nutrition you need to stay healthy long-term. Due to seasonal availability of food and soil depletion, you might want to consider the option of a high-quality multivitamin, though it's a good idea to talk to your doctor or a nutritionist to decide what's best for you.

Focus on Quality

There's no need to obsess over your food or eliminate everything that could be even remotely harmful from your life forever. Instead of creating stress and anxiety around your food, begin thinking more about quality, and the rest will take care of itself.

Portion Control

As much as this entire book focused on *what* you decide to eat instead of how much you eat, quantity does still matter, if only in regard to your budget.

One of the main arguments against buying organic food is the price tag associated with it. When you set your sights on quality, you have the ability to eat less and enjoy your food and your health more.

High-quality food is more nutrient-dense, which not only means more vitamins and minerals working to keep you healthy, but it also means that each calorie you consume actually makes you feel full.

Empty calories aren't just devoid of nutrition; they're devoid of satiation. In order to fill up, you need to eat more, and more and then some more. While you're trying to fuel your body, you're creating the very hormonal imbalances that brought you to this book in the first place.

You don't have to diet for the rest of your life to maintain a healthy weight and feel great. But you do have to eat with your health in mind.

The nutritional value of organic food is much higher than industrially produced foods, and it doesn't come with the toxins, chemicals, and heavy metals that add insult to injury.

If you return to eating like you used to, you will have taken one very smart step forward only to follow it with hundreds of forkful sized steps backward.

When it comes to price, the major player is organic, hormone-free, pasture-raised meat, and dairy. If you're still concerned about the price, consider eating meat not just in smaller portions, but less frequently in your meals.

You just went 21 days without it; there's no reason you can go a few days a week without out for the rest of your life. Supplementing with high-quality organic legumes, pulses, soy, and certain grains and seeds can drastically cut the overall price of protein in your grocery bill.

At the same time, you'll be adding variety to your meals that will not just be exciting and delicious, but give you a more inclusive nutrient profile as well.

Finally, the more you–and everyone else in the world–buys organic, pasture-raised meat and dairy, the more the food industry will take notice. It's called voting with your wallet, and it works. The government currently subsidizes factory farms, but if demand shifts, so will their subsidies.

Go ahead and share this book with all your friends and family members. Hopefully, you'll be helping to improve their health as well as lower the costs of high-quality food in the long term.

The same is true for organic produce. Supply will follow demand, so choose organic at every opportunity and say no to the pollutants that are killing not just your body, but the entire world as well.

Invest in Your Health

It's not just the food that you're eating that you need to improve, but also the environment that you're living in. Everything from the air you breathe, to the water you drink and the products you put on your skin, has an impact on your health.

We've discussed environmental toxins in plastics and heavy metals. Invest in your health by buying long-lasting, high-quality food storage containers made out of glass or stainless steel. Avoid "non-stick" pans that leave slivers of chemical-laden materials in your food and invest in great stainless steel or cast iron pan. Products like this will cost more upfront, but they will last longer and be safer for you. In the long-term, it's an investment that makes sense.

You can also consider investing in a professional water filtration system for your home. Again, it comes with an upfront cost, but it will save you over time from buying either bottled water, which may not be any better for your health after all or disposable filters.

By filtering the water for your entire home, you're also protecting yourself from the chemicals and toxins in the water that you cook with and shower in.

Your skin absorbs everything it comes into contact with, including the water you wash with and the products you use to clean yourself with. Invest in your beauty products just like you invest in your food. Everything you put on your skin makes its way into your bloodstream just as surely as if you put it in your mouth and swallowed.

Take the mindset of "quality over quantity" into your life at large and let it rule your shopping habits from here on out. You and your health are worth investing in.

Chapter 11:

Physical Fitness is Always Helpful

Weight gain and retention is certainly not just about eating less and exercising more, contrary to popular opinion. But that doesn't mean physical activity isn't absolutely essential to your health.

You've heard the saying, "use it or lose it," and that couldn't be truer when it comes to your muscles and bones. Your muscles aren't just vanity features. Everything in your body operates because of muscle activity, and if you aren't moving your body on a regular basis, there will come a time when you won't be able to move your body at all.

If you're new to exercise, or if you're trying a new activity, working with a fitness professional who has a background in women's health and/or nutrition, health, and hormones can be a huge benefit.

Fitness During the 21-Day Diet

After reading this far into the book, you should be convinced that weight loss is not always about calories in versus calories out. Sometimes, your hormones make all the difference to your efforts.

When your metabolism is dysregulated and slow, exercise doesn't play as big of a role in weight loss as it would in a well-balanced body. *What* you fuel your body with is mainly responsible for weight loss success, or failure, but exercise does still make a difference.

Moving your body plays a role in balancing your hormones, so physical movement should be a part of your program right from the start. The type and intensity of activities you commit to will progress as you move forward in the reset.

Start Slow

Unless you're already an athlete, you should start slow. For the first few days, or even the first week, make it your goal to sit less simply– at least 90 minutes less if possible.

Ninety minutes add up quickly when you break up down into smaller stints. In an eight-hour workday, if you get up to walk around for five minutes every hour, you'll already have accounted for 40 minutes.

Depending on your own unique circumstance, you might consider using a standing desk, pacing around your office while you're on the phone, or simply drinking lots of water to give you a great excuse to have to walk to the bathroom every hour.

Since you'll be cooking more often, keep in mind that time spent chopping vegetables and sauteing fish is more physically taxing that time spent driving to a restaurant or ordering food from your computer.

If you've gone through your entire day and realize you didn't have a chance to move your body at all, instead of sitting down to watch an hour of television after dinner, cut it back to half an hour and spend the other time strolling around the block with your significant other, pet, or just your inner self.

It is a good idea to choose a time of day when you will be able to dedicate 20 - 30 minutes to exercise in the long term. You don't have to start out by training for a marathon or weight lifting competition, but simply getting used to a set time of day that is dedicated to movement is a good habit-forming base that will be helpful when you're ready to step up the intensity.

Increase Intensity

During the Insulin Reset, it can really help to burn off some glucose daily. Adding a short interval or burst into your current routine can be a great opportunity to get you accustomed to stepping up the intensity without adding a lot of stress to your workout commitment.

For example, if you've been going for an after-dinner walk for 30 minutes each evening, add a few sprints. Walk leisurely for five minutes, jog for 30 seconds, walk briskly for five more minutes, run for 30 seconds, walk briskly for five more minutes, sprint for 30 seconds, etc. This is a slow introduction to interval training that has been shown to improve insulin sensitivity and raise growth hormone greatly.

By the time you've successfully hit the leptin reset, your metabolism will be ready to start putting exercise to proper use in your weight loss efforts. When you first start to increase the intensity, focus on healing your body through stress-relieving activities, and realignment focused movements.

Start by being more intentional about your physical movements. Speed walking, hiking, or jogging out in nature are great stress relievers and easy ways to build up your endurance safely. You can also try swimming or bike riding.

Movements that realign your skeletal and modulatory body will also help realign your organs and digestive system, making your internal processes more effective. Practices such as yoga, Pilates, or barre class are great ways to step up the intensity of your fitness efforts in a safe, controlled, and restorative manner.

Above all, be safe. Work with a personal trainer if you're new to fitness, at least to get you started so that a) you'll be monitored and b) you'll learn the correct postures, positions, and movements, so you don't accidentally hurt yourself.

Fitness after the 21-Day Diet

Once your hormones are reset, you'll be ready to start focusing on other areas of health in your life, including your fitness. The reset focused primarily on your diet because the research shows that weight loss is primarily determined by what you put on your fork.

Making sure the weight stays gone, however, can be heavily influenced by your physical activity levels.

Exercise is an important component not just in your future hormone health, but in helping you stay youthful, strong, and energetic no matter what your age.

Depending on where your fitness levels are right now, you'll want to continue adjusting the intensity of your fitness upward as you get stronger and more fit. When it comes to exercise, it's always better to play it safe and work your way up gradually.

There are two forms of exercise that have been shown to improve hormonal health, and they also have anti-aging results: High-Intensity Interval Training (HIIT) and resistance or weight training.

Interval Training and Yoga

For many years, we've been told that if you want to lose weight, you have to do cardio. Lots of cardio. Science, not to mention millions of women worldwide who continue to lose weight on the treadmill, is finally telling a different story.

High-Intensity Interval Training (HIIT) is ideal in so many ways. First of all, it allows you to get an entire workout completed in only 20 - 30 minutes. It boosts the production of human growth hormone, which helps to stimulate fat loss and lean muscle production, and it doesn't overstress your body like endurance training can, causing a spike in your cortisol levels.

HIIT is simple and variable. You can apply it to nearly any type of exercise you enjoy the most, whether that's jogging, riding your bike, swimming or dancing. The goal is simple: add 30-second sprints of high intensity that push you past your comfort zone and require about 80% of your maximum heart rate.

Follow the sprints with a recovery period of around 40% of your maximum heart rate for 10 seconds and repeat the process three times for a total of three minutes. Once you've done one set, rest for two minutes, and then switch up the intervals for another three minutes session. Do this five times, and you've accomplished a very effective workout in only 25 minutes.

You only need to do this 25-minute work out three times a week to see better results that you experience running for hours a week on a treadmill.

To give your body the best stress-reducing recovery possible, you can incorporate yoga into your HIIT practice. Yoga is known as a relaxing, somewhat meditative activity that is wonderful for aligning your body and increasing zen. This is all true and very beneficial, but yoga and also work up a good sweat and create some beautiful, lean muscles.

To work it into your HIIT routine, do 30-second bursts of high-intensity bodyweight movements in between your yoga poses. Some great examples are mountain climbers, burpees, high knee sprints, jumping ropes, or ice skaters.

Resistance or Weight Training

Resistance training and weight training both focus on building muscle, and both have incredible benefits for your overall health.

Muscle is built through a natural process of damage and repair. Your body has a response dedicated specifically to helping you repair microtears in your muscles so that they grow stronger over time. It is natural and healthy.

Resistance training, as you might be able to guess, uses resistance to challenge your muscles, such as body weight or rowing a boat through the water.

Weight training, on the other hand, uses either free weights or weight machines to challenge your muscles beyond their normal use. For example, doing a bicep curl with an empty hand is going to provide you with very limited muscle usage, but if you lift a five or 10-pound weight, you'll be taxing your muscles.

In terms of helping you lose weight and keep it off when you focus on weight training, you get the benefits of what's called "afterburn." Because you've created damage to your muscles and stimulated your internal repair process, your metabolism also speeds up in order to fuel this extra repair process. This boost to your metabolism can burn additional energy for anywhere between 4 - 8 hours.

Building muscles puts stress on your muscles, but not necessarily on the rest of your body. This means you can enjoy the positive effects of a great workout without the downsides of increasing cortisol, provided you don't overextend your limits.

This is great news for women because it means not only do you never have to worry about bulking up, but you also can stick to shorter workouts, saving you time.

For best fitness results after your hormone reset, work your way up to three 20 - 30 minute HIIT workouts a week, incorporating yoga if you can, and two 30 minute resistance or weight training workouts.

Remember to enlist the services of a professional whenever you're learning new movements or routines. There are no benefits to hurting yourself while trying to improve your health.

Find the Right Fitness for You

How you exercise when you're 20 probably looks a lot different from how you will exercise when your 50 or even 80 years old. And it should.

At different stages of your life, your body needs different kinds of support.

When you're young and nimble, you can challenge your body in unique ways with less risk of injury. This is a great time to experiment and see what types of activity make you feel great and keep your interest. Setting a good foundation of cardio, strength training, and flexibility work will help you move through life in good condition.

Playing against your strengths will help you keep balanced. For women, this is more likely to look like weight training, whereas men might focus more on flexibility.

When you hit your mid-30s, your metabolism shifts, and with it, so should your exercise patterns. You might have to work a little harder to keep the weight from packing on and struggle a little bit more with the recovery time.

Did someone mention time? You probably have less of it to devote to exercise at this point in your life, so resistance training and high-intensity interval training (HIIT) will give you the best results in the shortest period of time.

Both those activities will also help you be proactive about bone health and muscle loss.

As you continue to age into your 40s and 50s, your fitness focus should be on maintaining your muscle mass and protecting your bones. Strength training and resistance exercises that also incorporate mobility and flexibility movements are perfect for this age group.

Consider activities like bodyweight based interval training, hiking, and Pilates.

Fitness in your 60s and beyond will depend heavily on your condition going into them. If you're already fit, continue doing what is working for you, but move toward lower-impact activities that still protect your bones and encourage muscle retention. If you're a runner, consider spending some time in swimming pools instead as needed.

You need to pay attention to your focus, controlling your movements carefully, and ensuring you are always stable and protected.

Have Fun

Exercise shouldn't be a punishment. It should be a reward. Life is hard, and moving your body should be fun, making you feel young and energetic again. Think about the happiest kids you've ever seen. What makes them so joyful? Running around, playing sports, and having fun.

If you can find a fitness routine that you enjoy and look forward to, you'll be much more likely to find a way to work exercise into your life. If you dread the thought of having to exercise, you might just give up before you even give yourself a chance to get stronger.

If you're new to fitness, take some time to experiment with different options.

Join a gym, take some classes, hire a personal trainer for a few weeks. You may find that group activities keep you motivated and help you enjoy your workouts. Or maybe beating your personal bests in a competition against yourself is what keeps you going.

You may find that working out inside, in a structured environment, makes you feel safe and focused, or an outdoor boot camp might get your heart racing with excitement.

Don't feel like there's only one way to stay fit. There are thousands of options for you to move your body, and finding the right choice for you is an individual decision.

Don't Hurt Yourself

The absolute most important factor in fitness is not to hurt yourself. Whether you're new to fitness or you've just been given a new burst of energy thanks to the hormone reset, it's important that you start at a level that is appropriate for your current state.

Jumping in too far too fast can end up in injury, and the last thing you want is another excuse to let your health and fitness degenerate.

Working with a professional and taking your time in any new fitness routine will help ensure you're able to continue moving your body every day for the rest of your life.

Conclusion

Life is much too valuable to waste feeling tired, weak, and in pain. Your body was meant to be full of energy, vitality, and get up and go. It's time you got that feeling back and held onto it for life.

This isn't about what the number on the scale says. That's just a byproduct. The more fantastic you feel, the better that number is going to look to you.

We live in a world that puts a lot of emphasis on size, clothes, and the current standards of beauty. The problem with those standards is that it's not really the size of the clothes the women in the magazine are wearing that you envy. It's their smile.

It's the implication that the beautiful women of the world are happy that makes the rest of the women in the world want to be like them. Women of the world have been struggling for decades to look like the women on the cover of magazines, even knowing that nothing about those standards are natural or even attainable.

It's time to stop killing yourself for the byproduct of what you really want, and start working toward the real goal: health and happiness.

Eating less and exercising more isn't going to bring you joy. It's probably not even going to change the numbers on the scale very much. It will make you miserable, though, if you work at it hard enough.

There is a better way.

Instead of punishing your body for damage beyond its control, you can start to appreciate it for all the hard work it does. You can nourish it and treat it with the love and constant devotion that it deserves. That you deserve.

Resetting your hormones isn't just about helping you lose weight. It's about guiding you toward life-long health that lets you live life to the fullest, enjoying every moment along the way.

An Effective Hormone Reset Diet

The recommendations outlined in this 21-Day Hormone Reset program are designed to help you get your metabolic system back in order by supporting your hormone-producing endocrine system.

The human body is remarkable. In as little as three days, your hormones can find their way back to homeostasis, provided nothing is confusing them or getting in their way.

Modern life is just as exciting and joyful as it is stressful, and balance needs to be addressed from all angles. Every decision you make throughout the day will affect your health, and the more you can trend toward health instead of away from it, the more you'll be able to enjoy all life has to offer.

By addressing the food you eat, removing items that cause disruption, and adding items that offer nourishment, you can support the systems of your body. A well-fueled body is designed to provide constant energy, stable moods, quick thinking, and unconscious weight management.

All the really hard work is done by your hormones. Your hormones are in charge of keeping your heart beating and your digestion moving. They protect you from disease and injury and brain damage.

In return, you feed them.

If you follow a Standard American Diet full of processed food, sugar, synthetic hormones, toxins, and heavy metals, you are feeding them poison.

On the other hand, if you feed them organic, natural proteins, fats, and plenty of vitamin and mineral-packed, plant-based carbohydrates, you'll be protecting and healing them just as surely as they protect and heal you.

Everything in nature follows a cycle. You get what you put in. Your body is very forgiving, and in as little as 21 days, you can see real health results. If you treat it like a crash diet, those results will fade just as quickly as your healthy habits do.

But if you change your lifestyle to support your health, these results can last a lifetime.

Sustaining Hormone Health for Life

Dieting is a thing of a modern, media-driven world, but it can be a thing of your past. None of them have ever worked for you before, or you wouldn't have read this book.

Calorie-based diets don't work in the long-term. Exercise obsessions are impractical and dangerous and, for most women, don't work either.

If you want to see a change in your body, a change in your health, you need to change how you treat your body. The Hormone Reset Diet is only a short, 21-day commitment to getting you started.

How you feel the rest of your life will depend on how committed to the changes, you are.

Do you want to wake up every morning feeling well-rested and ready to take on the day?

Would you love to be able to go on weekend adventures with friends and family, knowing that you not only have the energy, but you also can rely on your digestion to be on its best behavior?

Do you want to go out dancing, having the time of your life and fielding pick up lines all night long because you look so damn good, everyone in the room wants to get to know you better?

When you get hungry, would you like to reach for delicious food that you know is going to give you a better jolt of energy than the best double-espresso ever did? Do you want to impress your friends and family by feeding them "healthy" food that tastes better and is more satisfying than their favorite delivery?

Life is meant to be enjoyed. It's yours for the taking.

It won't always be easy, but it can be simple. You can stop agonizing over everything that has gone wrong in the past, and start appreciating everything that is ready to go right for you in the future.

The Hormone Reset Diet is just the beginning. You have the rest of your life ahead of you to feel this great and so much better.

Take care of yourself.

References

Biello, D. (2008, February 19). Plastic (Not) Fantastic: Food Containers Leach a Potentially Harmful Chemical [Web log post]. *Scientific American*. Retrieved September 18, 2019, from https://www.scientificamerican.com/article/plastic-not-fantastic-with-bisphenol-a/

Breastcancer.org. (2019). U.S. Breast Cancer Statistics. Retrieved September 13, 2019, from https://www.breastcancer.org/symptoms/understand_bc/statistics

Circadian rhythm. (n.d.). In Wikipedia. Retrieved September 17, 2019, from https://en.wikipedia.org/wiki/Circadian_rhythm

Foodprint.org. (2019). Antibiotics in Our Food System [Web log post]. Retrieved September 18, 2019, from https://foodprint.org/issues/antibiotics-in-our-food-system/

Gottfried, S. (n.d.). 15 Reasons To Rethink Red Meat [Web log post]. Retrieved September 13, 2019, from https://www.mindbodygreen.com/0-18145/15-reasons-to-rethink-red-meat.html

Gregor, M. [NutritionFacts.org] (2017, April 12). Are the BPA-free Alternatives Safe? [Video file]. Retrieved from https://youtu.be/QuMGcoEswTc

Qualiani, D,. Felt-Gunderson, P., (2017). Closing America's Fiber Intake Gap. *American Journal of Lifestyle Medicine*, 11(1), 80-85. doi: 10.1177/1559827615588079

Schwalfenberg, G. K. (2011, August 8). The Alkaline Diet: Is There Evidence That an Alkaline pH Diet Benefits Health? *Journal of Environmental and Public Health*. 2012. 7 pages. http://dx.doi.org/10.1155/2012/727630

Stachowicz, A. & Lebiedzinska, A. (2016, December). The effect of diet components on the level of cortisol. *European Food Research and Technology*. 242(12), 2001-2009. Retrieved from https://doi.org/10.1007/s00217-016-2772-3

Vanderpump, M. P. J. (2011, September). The epidemiology of thyroid disease. *British Medical Bulletin*, 99(1). 39–51. https://doi.org/10.1093/bmb/ldr030

Waldie, Paul. (2018, April 23). Protective mother wrestles lost polar bear. *The Globe And Mail Canada*. Retrieved from https://www.theglobeandmail.com/news/national/protective-mother-wrestles-lost-polar-bear/article703773/

Wellness Resources. (2008). The Leptin Diet: The 5 Rules of the Leptin Diet [Video File]. Retrieved from https://youtu.be/NwdxTRAH_Gs

Appendix 1: Meal Planning

The meals suggested in this section are not recipes, but rather guides to help you become more familiar with the foods that this reset encourages you to eat.

There are no quantities and no specific cooking times because each meal is designed to suit your own taste preferences. You can add variety in many ways, and each slight alteration will require a slightly different cooking time.

By using high quality, nutrient-dense ingredients and eating mindfully, your body will naturally tell you when it has had enough to eat, and counting calories shouldn't be necessary if you listen to your body's signals.

Get creative with the following meal suggestions and try to change up the ingredients every time you cook each dish to take in the most nutrients and minerals.

Breakfast Scramble

Starting your day with a healthy helping of clean, lean protein will help you maintain steady energy levels throughout the day, as well as kickstart your metabolism.

Since you'll be avoiding meat for the next 21 days, this breakfast scramble will provide you with plenty of options to mix and match proteins, as well as vary the other ingredients. With a little creativity, you can have a unique breakfast every day.

Ingredients

Start with your protein. Choose one of the following to be your base:

- organic, pasture-raised eggs
- organic tofu
- organic tempeh
- lentils
- quinoa

Add your healthy fats. Choose one of the following to saute your scramble:

- Extra Virgin Olive Oil

- Avocado Oil

- Coconut Oil

- Organic Ghee

You can also add some fresh avocado once your scramble is cooked. You don't need much oil, and always keep in mind that it's highly concentrated, so a little goes a long way. Eggs and soy-based proteins also have healthy fats in them, in a nature-intended balance of protein to fat.

Finally, add your carbs in the form of vegetables.

- at least one leafy greens, such as spinach, kale, orchard

- 2 - 3 other colorful veggies, such as broccoli, bell peppers, asparagus, zucchini, mushrooms, hot peppers

Lentils and quinoa are also high in carbohydrates, but we're not trying to focus on calories or macros. We're focusing on the quality and types of ingredients, making sure that what you're taking in supports optimal hormone production and regulation.

You can also add herbs and spices to flavor your scramble. Choose from any of the following or add your own personal favorites to the list:

- onion
- garlic
- basil
- rosemary
- cayenne

Try to choose fresh herbs when possible or dried herbs if you must. Avoid anything packed in oil or combined into a preformulated mix. Check the ingredients list to make sure the only thing listed is the herb you're planning on eating.

Directions

If you're using eggs, beat them raw in a bowl first. If you're using quinoa or lentils, have it pre-cooked and cooled. For a scramble made with tofu, crumble firm or extra firm tofu directly into a pan. Tempeh won't necessarily crumble, but you can break or cut it into small chunks.

Add your protein, oils, and finely chopped onion, if you're using it, to a pan on medium heat and start to sauté your scramble.

After a few minutes, add your chopped veggies and continue to mix everything until the vegetables are nicely cooked but not too soft.

If you're using garlic or other herbs, add them last, when there are only 2 minutes left to the cooking process.

Buddha Bowls

One of the most common signs of insulin resistance is constant hunger and the feeling that you need to eat every few hours. This is not ideal for survival or your hormones, so your new eating plan goal is to provide your body with enough sustainable energy to get you through four to five hours between meals.

Eating sufficient high-quality protein and healthy fats will help. You should already be eating protein-packed breakfasts, thanks to the Estrogen Reset Breakfast Scrambles, so now it's time to focus on your lunch, which can be more difficult to work protein into without relying on processed meats.

Buddha bowls have been popularized in recent years as vegetarian and vegan lifestyles have grown in popularity, and they're a great lunch option. They can be made ahead of time, focus on high quality, clean proteins, and incorporate healthy, low glycemic carbs and delicious fats.

They're also versatile enough that you can enjoy a different bowl every day of the week to avoid boredom and expand your flavor horizon.

Ingredients

Choose one of the following to be your protein-packed base:

- quinoa
- wild or brown rice
- cooked lentils or black beans

Add an extra protein (optional & pre-cooked):

- roasted chickpeas
- spiced lentils
- lightly fried organic tofu or tempeh
- shredded, boiled organic, pasture-raised chicken or turkey
- hard-boiled organic, pasture-raised egg

Add your vegetables (at least 3):

- fresh leafy greens like spinach, arugula, or watercress
- crispy raw veggies like cucumber, bell peppers, shredded carrots, shredded red cabbage, radish, broccoli sprouts

- steamed veggies like organic edamame,

- roasted veggies like sweet potatoes, broccoli, cauliflower, carrots, Brussels sprouts, squash

Get creative with fresh herbs

- fresh cilantro, basil, parsley, dill, or chives add fresh bursts of flavor

Finalize with healthy fats:

- Fresh avocado

- Raw nuts and seeds

- Homemade dressings, like tahini, peanut sauce or pesto

Bonus: fermented foods

- naturally fermented foods like sauerkraut, kimchi, miso, or some pickled veggies are powerful probiotics, great for gut health and full of intense flavor

Directions

Cook your base and proteins ahead of time so that you have them ready to incorporate into a bowl in a moment's notice. If you're going to cook any vegetables, have those pre-cooked as well.

To prepare your meal, get a large bowl or glass Tupperware container if you're bringing it to go.

Start with your base, using 2/3 – 1 cup of cooked quinoa, lentils, beans, or rice per serving. Add a small portion, about the size of your fist, of your prepared additional proteins. Add plenty of vegetables and herbs as much as you can eat. Decorate with any fermented foods, nuts, or seeds you'd like to add.

Finally, add your dressing when you're ready to eat.

This is a filling meal, so you won't be hungry again quickly, but the fresh vegetables will provide you with steady energy, and the healthy fats will make sure your brain powers you through the rest of the day. If this is your lunch, you don't have to worry about the mid-afternoon slump.

Super Soup

Soups are an amazing way to pack a lot of nutrition into a single meal and, if you're dealing with picky eaters, you can easily hide a wide variety of vegetables simply by pureeing them before adding them to the soup.

Ingredients

Choose one or a combination for your soup base:

- bone broth
- vegetable broth
- water plus stewed and pureed tomatoes

Add extra flavor to any of these options by sautéing onions, garlic, and celery in a small about of olive oil and then adding to your base.

Choose your protein:

- organic, pasture-raised chicken or turkey
- wild or brown rice
- lentils, chickpeas or black beans
- quinoa

- organic tofu

You can also add nutritional yeast for a healthy burst of flavor that is also high in vitamins, minerals, and protein. It creates a nutty, slightly cheesy flavor.

Add your vegetables (at least 3):

- leafy greens like kale, chard, spinach, arugula, or beet greens
- cruciferous vegetables such as shredded cabbage, broccoli, cauliflower, bok choy, or Brussels sprouts
- root veggies like sweet potatoes, carrots, turnips, parsnips, beets, or fennel
- squashes, such as pumpkin, butternut, zucchini or summer squash

While you can leave squash in hearty, bite-sized cubes, pre-cooking and pureeing them make for a creamy, subtly sweet soup base.

Select fresh or dried herbs:

- rosemary, thyme, oregano, parsley and basil each play out very well in soup, but don't hesitate to experiment with your own favorites

Directions

The easiest way to make a big batch of soup is to use a slow cooker. Add all your ingredients in the morning before you go to work or get on with the business of your day and put it on low. A crockpot will be safe to leave on whether or not you're home, and will slowly simmer your soup to perfection over the next 6 – 8 hours.

If you don't have a slow cooker, you can add all your ingredients to a large stockpot and cook over medium to low heat for 1 – 3 hours, stirring occasionally.

You can cook soup quicker, if you are diligent in watching the stove and frequently stirring, allowing for a low boil.

Most soups freeze incredibly effectively, so making a large batch to save some for future quick meal solutions is a time and money-saving plan.

Stuffed Veggies

Many vegetables lend themselves very well to being stuffed. This is a great way to make a vitamin-packed vegetable the star of your meal, supported by the remaining ingredients. If you've become overly reliant on pasta and rice and you're struggling to make easy meals without these high-glycemic carbs, stuffed veggies are a creative alternative for dinner.

Ingredients

Vegetables that stuff well:

- bell peppers
- tomatoes
- acorn squash
- eggplant, zucchini or summer squash
- artichokes
- avocado
- portobello mushrooms

You can also use cabbage, collard greens, or other large green leaves to "wrap" your filling instead of getting stuffed.

Alternatively, baked potatoes and sweet potatoes can have their insides scooped out and mashed, added to the filling, and then stuffed.

Pick your protein (pre-cook):

- shredded, boiled organic, pasture-raised chicken or turkey
- crumbled organic tofu or tempeh
- lentils or black beans
- quinoa
- wild or brown rice
- organic edamame

Add your vegetables (at least 2):

- finely chopped fresh leafy greens like spinach, kale, arugula, beet greens or swiss chard
- finely cubed pieces of carrot, bell pepper, broccoli, cauliflower, and the edible centers of any vegetable you are planning on stuffing
- sautéed onion, garlic and/or celery for added flavor

Directions

Pre-cook your protein.

Clean and empty the center of the vegetable you have chosen to stuff. If you're using bell peppers, you can discard the seeds, but the centers of all the other options can be re-incorporated into the filling to avoid waste.

Combine your cooked protein and your vegetables together in a large bowl.

Fill your primary vegetables and roast in the oven for 20 – 40 minutes, depending on the vegetable you've chosen.

If you're stuffing a hearty squash, like acorn, you might want to pre-cook it halfway before stuffing it in order to avoid either undercooking the squash or overcooking the filling.

Spiced Chia Pudding

This incredibly easy to make dessert or meal replacement is high in protein, fiber, and, depending on your unique additions, flavor.

You can make it without sugar or dairy, making it a diabetic, gluten-free, vegan-friendly dessert that can be eaten in place of any meal without guilt.

Ingredients

The only two mandatory ingredients are:

- chia seeds
- milk or milk alternative

For the biggest health impact, choose organic, unsweetened options.

Depending on where you are in the reset and your own unique food sensitivities, you have a wide variety of added flavors that you can enhance your chia pudding with. The fruit is the most popular option, but it's not exclusive.

- Pureed fruit, such as pineapple, stewed apples, or berries

- Nut or seed butter

- Dark chocolate

- Fresh or dried coconut

Adding fresh or dried spices can also incorporate big flavor without the sugar-load pitfall. A few great combinations include:

- Cinnamon, nutmeg, cloves, allspice

- Ginger and turmeric, with a touch of cayenne

- Ginger and cinnamon

- Mint

Directions

To make your pudding, simply soak ¼ cup of chia seeds in 1 cup of milk or milk alternative for at least an hour, refrigerated.

When the chia has soaked up all the milk, you can add your pureed flavorings and spices. For a textured pudding, just mix in the additions, and for a smoother, more traditional pudding mouth feel, blend everything together.

Serve cooled.

AUTOPHAGY

How to Learn to Achieve a Healthy Lifestyle With Weight Loss Thanks to Intermittent Fasts, a Keto Diet, and Physical Activity

Alexander Phenix

Chapter 1:

Here Are the Processes and Paths

This chapter will explain what autophagy is, its pathways, and the most important types of autophagy:

- Macroautophagy
- Microautophagy
- Chaperone-mediated autophagy

What is autophagy?

The best starting point for understanding autophagy is its etymology. This term comes from the Greek words "auto" (self) and "phagein" (to eat), so the term is self-explanatory, it means to eat oneself. Well, there is a bit more than that to autophagy, this is why you will need to pay attention to the following lines. Autophagy represents the body's mechanism that gets rid of damaged or old cells and pieces of cells. These include things like cell membranes, organelles, and proteins when there isn't enough energy to preserve the damaged and old cell machinery, which happens to be composed of all these pieces just mentioned above. But that's not all! Autophagy is also the process of degrading and recycling various cellular components, but it can be so easily confused with apoptosis, as this is the process that schedules cell death. When you think of apoptosis, you can picture an old car, which doesn't even start, so you need to dispose of the old parts which are not functioning anymore. Therefore, apoptosis replaces old cells with brand new ones when the old cells are no longer working like they did when they were young. So yes, you can consider apoptosis your body's mechanic, capable of replacing the parts which are no longer working, with brand new ones, which work perfectly. But everything is done at a cellular level.

Autophagy, on the other hand, happens at a subcellular level and is responsible for destroying subcellular organelles, as well as for replacing or rebuilding new ones. The lysosome organelle is very important in the autophagy process because it has enzymes dedicated to degrading proteins from old cellular parts. Do you know what starts autophagy? The process is triggered by metabolic stress, like nutrient deprivation, growth factor depletion, and hypoxia. The principle is simple, every cell has to get rid of subcellular parts and recycle them (turning them) into new proteins, or just energy the cell needs to survive. Autophagy can be considered the housekeeper at a sub-cellular level, as it disposes of the old sub-cellular components and replaces them with new ones.

Autophagy has three main roles:

- Remove damaged proteins and organelles
- Avoid any abnormal protein aggregate accumulation
- Remove intracellular pathogens

Indeed, autophagy requires healthy cells to eat dead cells, so the healthy ones are looking for dead cells to consume when this process gets enabled. The autophagosome is the main referee of this process, as it represents an organelle capable of combining an endosome and lysosome to form a double membrane around the cell that's about to be consumed. This double membrane will dissolve the cell and convert it into energy. This can also be done on a smaller scale inside a cell to dissolve sub-cellular components. It's still not clear where the autophagosome originates, but it looks like it's formed when there are many proteins at the "pre-autophagosomal structure" (PAS).

In most cases, autophagy is triggered by nutrient starvation:

- In yeast, autophagy can be triggered by factors like nitrogen starvation or reductions in nucleic acids, carbon, auxotrophic amino acids, or even sulfate.
- When it comes to plant cells, autophagy can be triggered by carbon and nitrogen starvation.
- In mammals, autophagy can be induced in different tissues and in various degrees. It can occur in the liver, brain, muscle, or trigger mitophagy in a process called Chaperone-Mediated Autophagy (which we will talk about a bit later in this chapter). When the number of amino acids gets too low, this is a powerful signal that can activate autophagy, but it can also depend on the cell type and amino acids because amino acid metabolism may differ across different tissues.
- Another key player that can regulate autophagy is the endocrine system, especially insulin signaling. When blood sugar rises and indicates the presence of different nutrients, especially glucose, it completely crushes liver autophagy. There is a counterpart to insulin, called

glucagon, which is responsible for releasing glycogen from the liver to be used for energy, and this improves autophagy.

Usually, autophagy can be seen as a catabolic pathway that makes you destroy old cells. It leads to protein breakdown, but this process still requires muscle homeostasis. If autophagy is not functioning properly, you will be faced with a problem in maintaining lean tissue. Autophagy is also known for handling atrophy and catabolism a lot easier through protein austerity. You don't want your muscles to age or to waste away due to defective or excessive autophagy. Cells can be kept alive through mTOR and insulin (which are both anabolics), and this is one of the reasons why hardcore bodybuilders and athletes choose an anabolic lifestyle, just to prevent muscle catabolism. They focus on muscle growth by consuming protein supplements or different amino acids. However, keep in mind that autophagy will be suppressed if you always take nutrients and have access to energy constantly. But if all the macronutrients are not used to generate energy, this can lead to less responsive cells.

Autophagy plays a very important role in supporting the plasticity of your skeletal muscles as a response to endurance exercise. But if you want autophagy to be enabled during endurance exercise, AMPK (adenosine monophosphate-activated protein kinase) has to be triggered too since this is a very important enzyme involved in cellular energy homeostasis. This enzyme activates the uptake of glucose and fatty acids (and oxidation, too) when the cellular energy is low. Therefore, it's fair to say that AMPK can adjust protein synthesis and breakdown pathways. This enzyme can only be triggered through energy stress, nutrient deprivation, and tough exercise and will help create a protein called LC3B-II, which is important for autophagy. So, the best time to work out is when your body is in a fasted state because LC3B-II levels are higher and the body will go straight to the fat tissue for energy, and not to the nutrients you just had from your last meal. AMPK has a significant contribution to better oxidation of fatty acids, but it also improves glycolysis flux and prevents the synthesis of glucose, fatty acids, and cholesterol.

If you want to grow or repair your vital organs and muscles, your body will need to fluctuate from anabolism to catabolism since both of these states are very important for a healthy life. Nobody knows for sure when autophagy really happens, all that we know is that it can happen in different degrees most of the time (probably all of the time). In order to make autophagy happen, you will need to suppress mTOR and insulin, as this will significantly increase the chances of triggering autophagy. Lower liver glycogen and blood glucose can be signals of energy deficit in your body, and when the energy is getting lower, the body can trigger the metabolic pathways associated with burning the fat tissue for energy. This can lead to a higher ketone level in your blood, so your body is entering the state of ketosis. If you plan to keep your blood glucose and insulin level down, this strategy can help you maintain autophagy while the ketone levels are getting higher. Ketosis and autophagy usually go together, and in many situations, ketosis is the first phase of autophagy. However, this doesn't mean that ketosis will automatically trigger autophagy, as you can be in a ketosis state without activating autophagy. This is possible through nutrient signaling and mTOR, as it can still be activated by the consumption of large quantities of fats in the wrong circumstances.

Autophagy can start after 24 hours of fasting after your last meal (let's say that you follow a diet which is rich in carbs). I know this may sound too harsh, but if you want to experience all the benefits of autophagy, you may need to fast for at least 48 hours, thus giving your immune system and stem cells enough time to work their "magic" and do their "thing." Some specialists would highly recommend trying 3-5 days of fasting two or three times per year. Why? Because you will burn plenty of body fat, but you will also recycle weak cells, which can otherwise cause some issues. Our daily feeding habits, with three main meals per day, plenty of junk food (or other food rich in carbs), and a lot of snacks consumed is, in fact, the most common type of overconsumption, and will never lead to autophagy or recycling of old cells. In such a situation, you are overfeeding yourself, and you are not giving your body a chance to clean itself.

Types of Autophagy

Macroautophagy

Macroautophagy is responsible for the degradation of aggregated or misfolded proteins and dysfunctional organelles. It's simply a process that represents an important pathway for maintaining cellular homeostasis, especially in neurons (or other non-mitotic cells). Macroautophagy is all about the formation of autophagosomes and the collaboration between them and lysosomes. Now, you are probably wondering where autophagosomes form. They form in the cytoplasm from phagophores that will eventually consume parts of the cytoplasm filled with lipid substrates and proteins.

However, no one knows for sure the origin of the growing membrane. It can come from the plasma membrane, Golgi, endoplasmic reticulum, and mitochondria, as any of these sources can provide enough lipids for the growth of autophagosomal membranes. But only the fusion of autophagosomes with lysosomes can trigger the degradation of damaged cell parts within the membrane.

For a few central nervous system diseases, aging can be considered one of the biggest risk factors for their development and targets for their cure, but the mechanism behind this is still elusive. Macroautophagy plays an important role when it comes to neurodegenerative diseases like Alzheimer's or Parkinson's disease. Manipulating the levels of macroautophagy could be beneficial in various brain disorders, as discovered in the past few years in Alzheimer's disease and amyotrophic lateral sclerosis (ALS).

Macroautophagy impairment has been shown to have the opposite effect, as it was able to trigger the neurodegenerative process by itself, which supports the idea of therapeutic strategies targeting enhanced macroautophagy. This is why it is highly important that the macroautophagy process functions properly. Damaged organelles can be removed through processes like mitophagy, pexophagy, and ribophagy. Macroautophagy is often referred to as autophagy by many authors and specialists.

Microautophagy

This process is about moving particulate or soluble constituents into lysosomes. Microautophagy transfers cytoplasmic substances into lysosomes to be degraded through direct invagination, septation, or protrusion of the lysosomal limiting membrane. Nutrient deprivation is what triggers microautophagy, but it can also be launched by rapamycin or nitrogen starvation. This process is very useful for the maintenance of organelle size and the composition of the membrane in addition to its role in cell survival under nutrient deprivation.

The functions of microautophagy can be seen below:

- It can regulate the composition of the lysosomal/vacuolar membrane.
- It can deliver glycogen into lysosomes.
- It can consume multivesicular bodies that are made by endocytosis, so it has a very important role in the turnover of membrane proteins.
- It can maintain the composition of biological membranes and the size of organelles. It's also responsible for cell survival under nitrogen starvation and for aiding the transition pathway from starvation-induced growth to logarithmic growth.

The tests about non-selective microautophagy were mostly done in yeast, but the same molecular principles apply to every organism. There are a few different steps for this process, as seen below:

- Autophagic tube formation and membrane invagination
- Vesicle formation
- Vesicle expansion and fission
- Vesicle recycling and degradation

Chaperone-mediated Autophagy (CMA)

This represents one of the main pathways of autophagy, alongside macroautophagy and microautophagy. It's a more recent discovery, so probably some of you have never heard of it or have found out about it only recently. Intracellular proteins undergo coordinated synthesis, recycling, and degradation of their amino acids. They are subject to this continuous turnover process, which allows proper control over them and represents a way to regulate multiple intracellular processes. Proteins can be degraded through the action of lysosomes and proteasomes. In this process, they are targeted from the cytosol to the lysosomal membrane, but then they cross the membrane gaining access to the lumen of this organelle. This process is known as chaperone-mediated autophagy (CMA).

An interesting fact about CMA is that it selects proteins individually, so it has a regulatory role in different cellular processes by altering the intracellular levels of enzymes, cell maintenance proteins, and different transcription factors.

Now, let's try to understand how chaperone-mediated autophagy really works. The process has four different steps:

- Substrate recognition and lysosomal targeting
- Substrate binding and unfolding
- Substrate translocation into the lysosome
- Substrate degradation in the lysosomal lumen

Some of the main functions of CMA are:

- It recycles amino acids during prolonged starvation.
- It degrades regulatory metabolic enzymes, leading to adaptation of cancer cells to low nutrient conditions.
- It has an important role in quality control, and this is associated with the ability to remove single proteins from the cytosol.

Chaperone-mediated autophagy can be upregulated in other conditions leading to protein damage like exposure to denaturing toxic compounds. When triggered, CMA is also known to support the survival of retinal cells during the pro-apoptotic program. It looks like chaperone-mediated autophagy can be activated through hypoxia, and it's essential for cell survival.

Chapter 2:

What Could These Benefits of Autophagy Be?

I like to consider autophagy, a cellular housekeeper who has different roles like removing intracellular pathogens, defective organelles, and also damaged proteins (after all, we don't want abnormal proteins to accumulate). Some of the main advantages of inducing autophagy are the prevention of cancer, atherosclerosis, or other neurodegenerative diseases like Alzheimer's or Parkinson's disease. But there are a few more benefits to autophagy, so you can easily see how good this procedure is for your body. Autophagy has anti-aging effects within your body, as it can help destroy and recycle damaged parts occurring in spaces between cells and within cells. Therefore, the autophagy process can focus on using the waste produced inside cells in order to develop new "building materials" that can help with regeneration and repair.

The studies on autophagy are still in their early stages, so there are still many things to be discovered. However, so far, we know that it plays a key role in "cleaning up" the body, and also in protecting it from the negative effects of daily stress. Some of the most important benefits of autophagy are:

- It can generate molecular building blocks and energize cells.
- It can recycle organelles, aggregates, or damaged proteins.
- It can adjust the functions of the mitochondria within cells, and all of this can have a significant role in developing energy for the cell and can be influenced by aspects like oxidative stress.
- It can clear damaged endoplasmic reticulum and peroxisomes.
- It can protect the nervous system and encourage the growth of nerve and brain cells. Although it's still debatable, autophagy can improve neuroplasticity, cognitive function, and brain structure.
- It can prevent heart diseases and encourage the development of heart cells.
- It can eliminate intracellular pathogens and enhance the immune system.

- It defends the body from any toxic proteins that might contribute to amyloid diseases.
- It can protect the DNA's stability.
- It can prevent necrosis (which means the damage to healthy tissues or organs).
- It's known to prevent neurodegenerative diseases (Alzheimer's or Parkinson's disease), cancer, or other illnesses.

Autophagy studies were mainly conducted in microorganisms but have also been conducted in mammals (like mice or rats). It was clearly shown that autophagy could occur in any living organism, including humans. There are at least 32 autophagy genes, and perhaps science will discover even more of them. For plenty of species, autophagy can occur after stress and starvation (both symptoms can be induced through Intermittent Fasting and nutrient deprivation).

However, the benefits mentioned above don't stop there, as there is more. Since this process is induced through Intermittent Fasting, following a Keto Diet, or through really intensive training, autophagy will eventually lead to weight loss as well. Fatty cells are being destroyed, and they are replaced with muscles. Plus, it will always maintain the youth and strength of your cells, as this process also involves cellular rejuvenation.

I like to think that autophagy has the sum of all the benefits that come along with Intermittent Fasting, the keto diet, or physical exercise. All of them have plenty of health, physical, and psychological benefits, so why not try this process every 3 or 4 months? Since we are living in a world full of diseases, and most of them are caused by our eating habits, inducing autophagy can be the tool we have on hand to reverse the negative effects of our eating habits.

Most diets are only focused on losing weight, they are extremely harsh, and most people can't stick to them. However, how many of these diets can actually induce autophagy? Truth be told, only a few of them. The modern-day diets do not consider any health effects. They just focus on the weight loss process. Such programs don't include the autophagy process, so their health benefits are extremely limited. Since autophagy can be induced by nutrient deprivation (through Intermittent Fasting and the keto diet), or through extremely intense exercises (like HIIT), it's really hard to think of any other method that can have the same benefits of autophagy.

This is why, whenever you choose a diet, you need to do your homework first, just to make sure it can induce autophagy. Intermittent Fasting can work wonders for you, as it can be such a path to autophagy, while the keto diet is another one. But what if you combine them together? What if you combine Intermittent Fasting, Keto Diet, and HIIT (High-Intensity Interval Training)? In this case, you can only speed up and maximize the effects of autophagy. Therefore, you can try a daily fasting program (like the Leangains program, as seen in a future chapter of this book), have keto food in your feeding window, and work out extremely intensely in a fasted state. Just imagine the results you will have! It will not be easy; in fact, it will be extremely challenging, but all the benefits mentioned above should give you the extra motivation to aim for autophagy.

The older we get, the more damage we have throughout our body, which is something that immune receptors can easily acknowledge and encourage the production of plenty of pro-inflammatory molecules. When the accumulated damage is too great to be handled, inflammation becomes chronic, and this can lead to many age-related diseases.

In general, inflammation can't be considered a bad thing (keep in mind that acute inflammation is part of the healing process), but chronic inflammation can easily be associated with poor health biomarkers. Nutrient deprivation can trigger plenty of mechanisms, but it also constrains nuclear factor-kB (NF-kB), which has an anti-inflammatory effect. NF-kB can be considered one of the master regulators of inflammation as it decreases its activity and plays an important role in downregulating many aspects of pro-inflammatory signaling.

Chapter 3:

Its Own Function

This chapter is for understanding how autophagy functions, how it's induced, and what its actions are. I will try to spare you the very complicated medical terms and to explain in words everybody can understand. After all, autophagy should be more popular and should be understood by the wide majority of people.

Nutrient Starvation

Nutrient starvation is just one of the ways to trigger autophagy, and it can be done through Intermittent Fasting or a proper keto diet. The process of autophagy is not something that can happen just like that, as much as we would like to do it. It needs to be induced, and starvation is one of the ways to achieve it. During autophagy, you are getting rid of damaged cell parts, organelles, or toxic proteins, but this process can't happen when you are overfeeding yourself.

Intermittent Fasting is a process of nutrient deprivation and meal scheduling (if you are doing it on a daily basis). In Intermittent Fasting, you significantly cut down on the calories you consume since you skip at least one meal per day, the goal of which is to induce nutrient starvation. Your body is not used to fasting; it's probably used to eating on a regular basis, to having three main meals per day, and perhaps even some snacks are few times per day. In this case, you are consuming a lot of calories, which will never be burned. The calories you consume are in the form of carbs (glucose), and since the glucose is never fully consumed, it gets stored in your blood, raising your blood sugar level. Now, you are probably aware of what will happen if the blood sugar keeps rising, but this will need to be discussed in another chapter of this book.

The main purpose of Intermittent Fasting is to get the body into the fat-adapted phase through nutrient deprivation. We all like to think that a properly balanced meal or daily meal plan should have around 40% protein, about the same carbs, and only 20% fats. Now let's start with proteins! Everybody knows that there are a number of proteins required just to maintain muscle mass, but it is highly unlikely that you will be able to maintain a ratio close to 40%

protein in your total nutrient intake (not even if you stuff your face with protein bars or drink a lot of protein shakes). Pure proteins in food are not that easy to be found, and as much as we need them, the chances are low that you will get that much protein in your meals. Bear in mind that physical exercises are what can grow your muscle mass (although its true this is enhanced by serious protein intake). Otherwise, all your protein consumption would be in vain when it comes to building muscle mass. Proteins are just the nutrients required to maintain your muscle mass or to help build it.

Paradoxically, Intermittent Fasting has shown a way to grow your muscle mass, even when you do not have any proteins or nutrients at all. It looks like experiencing days of complete fasting (no calories whatsoever) can stimulate your growth hormone production like nothing else; this is why its level goes through the roof after 48 hours of fasting. When on an Intermittent Fasting program, you can reduce your calorie intake on a daily basis, or you can go for days without eating anything. Your body enters the autophagy phase after 24 hours of fasting (by fasting, I mean no calories at all).

Since your body is already so used to running on glucose, it will not switch immediately to fats when it runs out of glucose. Ketones will provide energy for a short time when your body is in ketosis metabolic state, but by the time your body reaches the autophagy phase, it should already be running on fats. Low insulin and glucose levels can be compensated for by higher ketones levels, and this is why your body is such a wonderful "machine" because it can easily adapt to all situations, including nutrient deprivation.

If you think about it, only good things can come if you let your body run on fats, since you are literally breaking down the fat tissue to burn fat and release the energy (and also removing the toxins stored in your fat tissue that can affect your internal organs). However, nutrient deprivation doesn't have to mean any calories at all. It can also be radically changing your diet and removing (or almost completely removing) one macronutrient. I'm talking about carbohydrates, the main source of our health problems generated by improper feeding. It doesn't come as a shock that we are all eating so much, drinking a lot of sweet stuff, and accumulating a lot of carbs and sugar in our bodies. We are aware of this issue, but we are still eating and drinking the same "garbage" over and over again.

Probably most of us are not aware of what healthy food looks like or simply can't afford it. The biggest problem is that carbs are causing addiction. You can never consider most food types containing carbs to be satiable and consistent enough. These food types are indeed caloric bombs, but it seems that they only focus on quantity, not on quality. Soon after you had your meal, you will feel hungry again, and your body will crave more carbs. This is the time when you are stuffing your face with snacks (chips, donuts, chocolate bars, and other kinds of sweets). Therefore, it's a vicious circle, as once you are hooked on carbs, then your body will crave more carbs, over and over again.

Getting out of this vicious cycle can be extremely difficult, but Intermittent Fasting can do the trick along with the keto diet. The trick is to train your body to run on something other than glucose to make it run on fats. Not only IF can do that for you, but also the keto diet. For those of you not familiar with this term, a ketogenic diet is an LCHF (low carbs high fats) meal plan designed to replace the excessive amount of carbs from your standard diet with fats. Yup! You've heard me right! Eating fats can be healthy for you, as it can switch your body's energy source from glucose to fats. Energy is provided by ketones in the transition period when there is no more glucose, and the body is desperately looking for an alternative and sustainable energy source. Therefore, ketones (the chemical compounds responsible for the metabolic state of ketosis and for naming the keto diet) can be considered the "backup generator" for your body. What can be more reliable and sustainable than the energy source provided by your fat tissue? You already have it stored in there, and through the keto diet, you are refueling your body with fat, so it runs on this energy source.

This diet significantly lowers your carb intake, or perhaps even eliminates any source of carbs from your daily menu, so your body is no longer receiving glucose. Therefore, you are not confusing your body, and you let it run on fats. Who would have thought that eating fats can get you thin? Of course, you will need to plan the size of your meals carefully, but you can actually achieve this if you lower the calorie intake per meal. You can't expect to stuff your fats with fats, eat plenty of calories, and lose a lot of weight. This won't happen! Instead, if you measure your portions, you can achieve the goals that you want: you can lose weight and induce autophagy as well. It's not an exact science, so no one knows for sure the time required to reach the autophagy phase through a keto diet. All that we know is that you will eventually get there.

Xenophagy

Xenophagy represents a radical change of diet, like a carnivore becoming a herbivore, but from a microbiological point of view, it represents the autophagic degradation of infectious particles. In this process, intracellular pathogens like viruses, protozoans, or bacteria that are all inside the cytosol (inside the cell membrane) or in some pathogen-containing vacuoles covered by isolation membranes, are simply consumed into autophagosomes and degraded inside autolysosomes.

Therefore, not only does autophagy function in adaptive and elemental immunity, but there are also some mediators involved in the intracellular pathogens that can control and stimulate autophagy. Out of these mediators, we can include the interferon-inducible antiviral molecule PKR, as well as CD40-CD40 ligand interactions, TNF-alpha, T-helper type 1 lymphocytes, the cell surface receptor TLR4, IFN-Y, and its immunity-related GTPases. The vacuoles (spaces) used to engulf intracytoplasmic bacteria are quite similar to autophagosomes, but their formation also requires autophagy.

But let's stopover here with the fancy medical terms. Autophagy is not possible without xenophagy, as a radical change needs to happen in our daily menu. Whether we are not consuming any calories, or we are just cutting down (almost completely) on carbs. The food we eat provides the energy source for our daily tasks. Now, as you already know, burning calories produces energy, which must be consumed. This is why you need to efficiently feed yourself, as you don't want too much glucose in your system. Preferably, you will not store any glucose at all in your blood, but this is up to what you eat and how much exercise you are doing on a daily basis.

So far, there aren't any studies to show that fats as an energy source are lower quality than the glucose energy source. So, you are not switching to a lower quality "fuel type." The best part about fats is that the fat reserves are already there; they are stored in your body. This is what makes this energy source more sustainable. It can also be considered a "green" source of energy, as there are some toxins stored in your fat tissue, and breaking the fat tissue for energy will automatically eliminate the toxins as well.

If you stick to glucose as your energy source, then autophagy will simply not happen unless you train at an extremely intense level to eliminate all of your glucose stored in your body and blood. Since this is highly unlikely, xenophagy needs to happen in order for autophagy to be induced.

Infection

Infection is just one of the functions that can trigger autophagy. Autophagosomes can take vesicular stomatitis virus from the cytosol and move it to the endosomes, where it can be detected by the toll-like receptor 7 (pattern recognition receptor), which can detect single-stranded RNA. After the toll-like receptor has been triggered, intracellular signaling cascades are initiated, and this can lead to the induction of different antiviral cytokines or interferon production. Some bacteria and viruses can subvert the autophagic pathway and are capable of promoting their own replication. One of the recently discovered intracellular "danger receptors" is Galectin-8; this receptor is capable of initiating autophagy against intracellular pathogens. When it binds with a damaged vacuole, Galectin-8 can call up an autophagy adaptor like NDP52, and this can lead to bacterial degradation and the formation of the autophagosome.

Repair Mechanism

Autophagy acts at a cellular level, but its effects can be seen throughout the whole body. This process destroys damaged organelles, proteins, or cell membranes. When you think about it, these damaged parts are exactly what's causing aging to progress at a faster pace. Now let's get something straight! Autophagy is not the "fountain of youth" as it can not freeze the aging process or reverse it. Humankind has yet to discover the cure for aging. Autophagy and its regulators can significantly slow down this process through its actions over the cells, as they are involved in response to lysosomal damage, often being steered by galectins like galectin-3 and galectin-8, which can recruit different receptors like NDP52 or TRIM16.

You are probably already lost in these terms. The bottom line which you need to remember when you are going through this process is that autophagy is responsible for destroying and recycling/replacing old or damaged cell parts like proteins, organelles, or cell membranes. This is why it can be thought of as a skilled mechanic that operates on an intracellular level.

Programmed Cell Death

Programmed cell death (PCD) can often be associated with the existence of autophagosomes and can also depend on autophagy proteins. As it turns out, this specific form of cell death can be considered autophagic PCD. The real mystery is whether the activity of autophagy over the dying cells is causing cell death or whether it is, in fact, an attempt to prevent it. There were a few studies trying to answer to this dilemma, but so far, there is no clear answer. So, at least at this point, we can't say that autophagy is the cause of programmed cell death, but there are some arguments stating that autophagy might, in fact, be a survival mechanism for the cell as it tries to prevent PCD.

Studies have been conducted on insects that clearly show a distinct form of programmed cell death, which involves autophagy. It looks like whether autophagy leads to lethality or survival can be easily distinguished by the degree or type of regulatory signaling during stress, especially after viral infection. These results may sound interesting, but so far, they haven't been tested on a non-viral system.

Chapter 4:

How Can We Behave Better by Applying Intermittent Fasting?

You probably don't know too much about fasting, or maybe you have only heard about it vaguely. When it's done for religious purposes, it's regarded as a purifying process, a process required for redemption, for the forgiveness of sins. Of course, you probably don't see the point in it, but there are religious fanatics out there who still practice it. Just think of the Ramadan period in the Muslim world!

Intermittent Fasting (or IF for short) is more of a self-discipline process which has plenty of benefits for human health. You are probably wondering what good can come out of starving yourself and not eating what you want. As it turns out, plenty of good things can come out of this practice. Keep in mind that this is not about starving yourself; it's about scheduling your meals properly.

Right from the beginning, you will need to properly understand two concepts: feeding (eating) window and fasting period. They are pretty self-explanatory, as they settle when to eat and when not to. Intermittent, by definition, is something that happens irregularly, and fasting represents a period during which you refrain yourself from eating. Putting it simply, Intermittent Fasting is a kind of lifestyle (that's right, lifestyle) that allows you to fluctuate from fasting to feeding periods properly.

Forget about all the very strict diets! They are only looking for immediate results, but as soon as you quit them, you will start gaining weight again. This is why IF is more of a lifestyle than a diet, as it involves a long-term commitment to yourself and to the feeding/fasting program. While most diets are after weight loss, this is only one of the numerous benefits you can get from following this plan. Unlike other diets, Intermittent Fasting doesn't come up with restrictions, so you can indulge yourself in every food you like, as long as you set a schedule and some rules.

This doesn't mean that you should stuff your face with junk food, as this type of food and any other low nutrition food should be avoided as much as possible during your feeding period.

That is if you want to maximize the results of Intermittent Fasting. Speaking of results, you need to set the right expectations, as this procedure will not guarantee you the best results in terms of weight and fat loss, but it can promise you the most consistent way to lose weight. You don't have to worry about gaining weight if you apply this procedure correctly and if you are in for the long run.

If you want to understand how IF works, you will need first to discover the role of the insulin. So, let's consider the regular diet of an average person, rich in carbs, junk-food, and snacks. During the feeding period, the glucose level goes up. This can only mean that the insulin level will skyrocket, and this can only prevent fat burning. Glucose is the default energy source of the human body, but in most cases, it's not fully consumed, so it gets stored in your blood, increasing the blood sugar level. High levels of insulin, typical for high glucose, can only mean "lazy" insulin, as it's not doing its job.

Probably most people would think that eating calories will automatically lead to more energy. Wrong! Consuming calories will release energy, not eating them. During your fasting period, as the hours go by, the insulin level lowers, favoring the fat burning process. It's believed that after 12 hours of fasting, the body is in optimal condition to burn fat, as glucose is no longer available, so the body will look for a different source of energy. Therefore, it will not burn the calories from glucose but instead will release energy after burning fat.

An extended fast period can only favor the fat burning process, but most people don't understand the meaning of fasting, so they extend the feeding window as much as possible during the day. The principle is simple. Most of the nutrients we consume are carbohydrates, the main source of glucose. High consumption of glucose will lead to a higher level of insulin, blocking the fat burning process, as the body will mainly use glucose for energy. This is the insulin-resistant state when too much insulin is secreted by the body. However, when this state becomes chronic, all the problems associated with the disease can start. You can expect low HDL, high triglycerides, abdominal fat storage, obesity, and eventually type 2 diabetes. Do you know how many people are in a pre-diabetes phase? About 35% of adults and 50% of elderly people are in this condition. Now, that's very frightening!

All of these people are constantly "re-fueling" with glucose, so they use it as the only energy source. This can only mean that they never had the chance of burning fat, as when they run out of glucose from their last meal, they will be starving for more and will eat again immediately. You can't expect your body to burn fat if it forgot how to mobilize fat for this process. This is why you will need to allow your body to burn fat. If you can refrain from eating for at least 12 hours, then you will train your body to go after your fat reserves for energy resources. Who said that you have to eat all the time just to have calories to burn? You can avoid eating (for a longer period) and focus on burning calories from your own fat reserves.

Now, of course, you will experience hunger, but are you willing to pay this price in order to burn fat? This is just at the beginning because as soon as you get used to the fasting process, hunger will no longer be an issue for you. Controlling hunger is Intermittent Fasting's main key to the fat-burning process. Feeding is a basic need of the human body, as it simply can't function properly without it. However, there are people who can go on for days without having anything to eat. Most people can go on for at least a week without food, but the current record is 382 days without food. This is a record set by a 456 pounds man who managed to lose 276 pounds during this period, without having any health problems after that. It should be noted that he conducted this fast under medical supervision and with the aid of vitamin and mineral supplements.

Starving yourself for so many days is definitely not recommended, so if you really have to fast for a very long period, you have to do it under the supervision of a physician. One of the main goals of Intermittent Fasting is to get the body into a fat-adapted state, which means using fat as the main "fuel." Now you are probably wondering: "Wait a minute! I'm fasting, and I'm not eating anything! How come the body uses fat as "fuel"? The body has the ability to break down its fat tissue and to release the energy stored there.

Do you want to burn more fat and to get your body into the right condition (fat-adapted state)? Then you better follow the simple rules listed below:

- Cut down on carbs, as they are preventing your body from transitioning into a fat-adapted state. You may need to consider an LCHF (Low Carbs High Fats) diet, which will lead to more fat burning since you are making your body run on fats.

- Physical exercise. You have all heard of the miracle diets of food types that will melt your fat away! Hint: this publicity stunt is just to catch your attention, as there is no better way to burn fat than physical exercise. As your body is being put through this type of activity, it needs to find the energy sources to carry on. This is why it will use the energy stored in your fat tissue.
- More calories don't necessarily mean more energy, so you have to be extremely careful with the number of calories you consume. More calories usually mean more glucose, so when you have lower calories, this can favor energy consumption from your fat reserves. Calorie watchers are usually shocked by the number of calories they can see on the label of each processed product. If you are wondering what to eat and what has fewer calories, the answer is very simple: natural and unprocessed food.
- Intermittent Fasting is a great way to prepare your body for the fat or weight loss process. This process can give plenty of chances for your body to burn fat, so the more you practice it, the more fat you will burn.

These are the golden rules if you want to lose weight. However, when you are fasting, it's important to avoid restricting your intake too much too fast. Don't starve yourself too much right from the beginning; this may cause serious discomfort, not just in terms of hunger but also in the form of headaches. This is why you need to ease into this process and to avoid rushing it.

If you are thinking of fasting, you will need to start with a plan that you can manage (you will find out more details about Intermittent Fasting plans in chapter 8 of this book). In other words, you need to start with a fasting period that you can easily cope with. Try 12 hours of fasting for starters, and then increase this period.

Hunger is something you can manage, but you need to get used to it first so you will not be too affected when you fast for longer periods. You might need to feed yourself a few times, just to get through the fasting period more easily, but the main point is to lower your food intake during the day and to stick to your feeding window. You may not be able to respect these rules in the beginning, but if you do, then kudos for you. This is what you should be aiming for, so it's up to you if you can stick with these rules. Intermittent Fasting is all about self-discipline and ambition. You need to set your own feeding and fasting periods, and you will need to stick to them. That's right! You shouldn't have any snacks during your fasting period (most of the time) if you want to maximize your results.

However, nobody said that you are not allowed to drink during your fasting period. In fact, this is highly recommended since your body needs the vitamins and minerals provided by water. You shouldn't have alcohol or juices for drinks, just stick to water, as this is the ideal drink you need to have. It doesn't have sugar, and it's the only type of drink that can calm your thirst, as all the other drinks will eventually make you even more thirsty. Obviously, you don't want to have soft drinks like Pepsi or Coca-Cola, as the amount of sugar is just too huge for the body to process. The excess of glucose will not do any good for your body.

You shouldn't have junk-food either! If you are a big fan of burgers, pizzas, French fries, and pasta, bear in mind that these types of food are the biggest sources of carbs. Cutting down on carbs is mandatory in such a situation. But what exactly can you eat? We are literally bombarded by processed food in which we can find most of the carbs we eat. We were told when growing up to eat our veggies. This couldn't be more applicable in this case. Therefore, you will need to let veggies have a bigger portion of your daily diet. If you look at the food pyramid, you will see that potatoes or rice have a higher concentration of carbs. This is why you will need to replace them with other veggies and any side dishes using these ingredients.

This is why you will need to have peas, beans, carrots, broccoli, cauliflower, and other vegetables in your daily menu. You don't have to become a vegetarian or a raw vegan, but you will need to have a properly balanced diet. Forget about your chips, chocolate bars, or other snacks that you used to have! There are plenty of carbs in these snacks, so they have to be ruled out. If you do want to try meat, make sure it's not processed. Grilled pork or beef can be OK, but sausages not. You will also have to be very careful with the quantities as well because you don't want to overdo it with meat.

Now, this sounds right, doesn't it! Eating healthy and alternating the feeding period with the fasting one. Obviously, if you are planning to practice Intermittent Fasting, then you will need to stay away from burgers, pizza, bread, rice, potatoes, pasta, and pastries. You probably think that there aren't too many options left. However, you couldn't be more wrong! You can have veggies, nuts, even meat (but in lower quantity). The main goal is to reduce the number of carbohydrates and also the number of calories.

The main features of our food are plenty of calories (very quantitative) and very low nutritional value (not too many nutrients other than carbs), so they are extremely low quality. You are probably wondering what to eat in order to cut down on carbs and replace them with something else. A very good alternative is the ketogenic (or for short, keto) diet. This is a type of LCHF (low carbs high fats) diet, which replaces the number of carbohydrates with a higher quantity of healthy fats.

The ideal nutritional percentage is very debatable, and it depends on the needs of every person. Obviously, a bodybuilder or an athlete needs more proteins, so their diet needs to have a higher percentage of proteins. Unfortunately, our daily diet has a very high percentage of carbohydrates. A keto diet is the exact opposite of a standard carb diet, as it lowers the carb level to less than 20% or even 15%. It fills in the gap with other nutrients like healthy fats and proteins (but mostly fats). Now here comes the paradox! How can you eat fats and lose them at the same time? Since you are training your body to run on fats, your body will burn fats, but if you are keeping the calories and quantities low enough, your body will consume more energy than you are eating, so it will go for the fat tissue.

What exactly can be considered a healthy fat? You can have olive oil, cheese, avocado, whole eggs, or different types of nuts. But, let's not spoil it for you, as the next chapter will be dedicated to this. If you are able to keep yourself in a fat-adapted state, then you are on the right path. This is why you can combine Intermittent Fasting with the keto diet. Obviously, you can choose the IF program which best suits your needs, but it's highly recommended that you tighten your feeding window (you can narrow it to less than 8 hours per day) and expand your fasting period. Although opinions can be different, there are plenty of nutritionists and specialists who believe that repeated fasting (so regularly alternating a fasting and feeding window) can be more effective than fasting for a longer period. The answer may be simple, as this way you can maximize the efficiency of your physical exercise, of your workout, while fasting for days will not guarantee you any efficiency when working out, as you feel powerless. Fasting for a very long period will give you headaches, and possibly stomach aches.

Therefore, remember to eat healthy food (following the keto diet is highly recommended) during your feeding period and to alternate your feeding and fasting periods. If you want even better results, don't forget to work out!

Benefits and Facts of Intermittent Fasting

There are a lot of reasons why you should try Intermittent Fasting, and below you can find just a few of the most important ones:

- It lowers oxidative stress and blood pressure.
- It enhances the fat-burning process.
- It speeds up your metabolism during the fasting period.
- It allows you to have better control over your appetite and blood sugar as well as enhancing your cardiovascular function.

Intermittent Fasting can be used for different reasons, as seen below:

- To burn fat
- To prevent disease

- Anti-aging effects
- Therapeutic benefits including physical, spiritual, psychological
- To increase mental performance
- To enhance physical fitness

There are plenty of specialists who state that there are eight main benefits of Intermittent Fasting:

- Destroying cancerous and precancerous cells
- Fostering a rapid shift into nutritional ketosis
- Lowering the fat reserves
- Enhancing gene expression for healthspan and longevity
- Enabling autophagy and apoptotic cellular repair/clearing (yes, autophagy is one of the main benefits of IF)
- Improving insulin sensitivity
- Lowering inflammation and oxidative stress
- Improving neuroprotection and cognitive effects

Intermittent Fasting for Weight Loss

Many people associate Intermittent Fasting with a diet, so they follow this procedure for weight loss. Shifting the energy source from glucose to fat cells is one of the main purposes of Intermittent Fasting, so when your body runs on fats, it literally burns fats, and you will notice your body getting thinner. Since you don't eat excessively, there aren't any chances of fat reserves building up, so when you consume fats, they will immediately get burned. However, your body still needs more; that's why it will go for your fat reserves.

Commitment is very important when you are following an Intermittent Fasting program. Not very many people stick to their diet, especially if the diet is too radical. IF it should be a lot easier to stick to, especially because it's not too restrictive in terms of what food you can eat. You can still eat anything you want, but there are some recommendations you should follow. Intermittent Fasting has a few phases, which include lipolysis, ketosis, and autophagy. All of these phases favor the fat loss process.

Intermittent Fasting for Disease Prevention

There are already plenty of studies showing the effect of Intermittent Fasting on blood glucose levels in diabetics. Obviously, when you train your body to quit carbs and glucose, the glucose level will decrease, and so will the insulin level. Funny fact! The insulin should regulate the blood sugar level, but when it's elevated to a very high level, it's simply not doing its job. But that's not all! There are other health benefits associated with Intermittent Fasting:

- It improves stress resistance.
- It significantly lowers inflammation and blood pressure levels.
- It improves lipid levels and glucose circulation, which can lead to a reduced risk of neurological diseases like Alzheimer's or Parkinson's disease, as well as cancer and heart diseases.

Intermittent Fasting for Anti-aging

As we already know, the modern-day lifestyle involves plenty of stress, junk food, and less rest. All of these factors can seriously impact the aging process. This is why we are experiencing signs of aging at earlier ages. This is a worldwide issue, so it's not specific to the western world. Humankind doesn't have the secret of long life or eternal youth. All people are subject to the aging process, but some of us experience this process a lot faster, while for others, this process goes a lot slower. Since it has an effect on the cells of your body, Intermittent Fasting can slow down the aging process since it goes after the main causes of it, plus it has an effect on cellular rejuvenation.

If you remember, autophagy is just the phase of Intermittent Fasting responsible for the self-detoxification process, during which damaged cells are being removed and replaced by new ones. When cells are replaced, this will impact the aging process, slowing it down for a while.

Intermittent Fasting for Better Mental Performance

We can say without any doubt that IF improves cognitive function, as it actually increased the power and functionality of the brain. These are not assumptions, as many people who went through a nutrient deprivation process have experienced a better concentration, a sharper mind, and better brain function. It may sound counterintuitive, but you can find better solutions to problems when you are going through nutrient starvation.

Nutrient deprivation triggers neural autophagy, a process that can lead to cell recycling or repair. Also, another positive fact of inducing neural autophagy is a higher level of BDNF (brain-derived neurotrophic factor), which is a protein activated by this procedure. BDNF is known for stimulating memory and also plays a role in cognitive and learning functions within the brain. It plays a major role in protecting the brain cells, and it also encourages the appearance of new ones. When your body is going into ketosis, ketones are feeding and energizing your brain, and this can lead to mental acuity and better productivity.

Intermittent Fasting for Therapeutic Benefits

This procedure can be used for therapeutic purposes, including psychological, spiritual, and physical improvements. Let's take them one by one and detail these kinds of benefits of Intermittent Fasting.

Psychological

Intermittent Fasting is a process of self-discipline, and it allows you to exercise your willpower and self-control. During the fasting period, you train your body not to eat anything, so you need a lot of ambition, just like when you are working hard at the gym. You are imposing on yourself the requirement to stay away from food during the fasting period, as well as when to eat or to control every aspect of your life.

Especially with women, but not only, IF can give you a better sense of achievement, pride, reward and of course, control. You will achieve improvements in self-esteem through this self-discipline process, which is considered one of the major predictors of success, happiness, and a better quality of life.

Spiritual

Fasting was practiced for a very long period of time for religious or spiritual purposes. It plays a role in penance and aims to aid in the redemption of sins. In Judaism, Christianity, and especially in Islam, fasting is practiced on a very wide scale. We all know about the Ramadan period, but this kind of fasting is way too radical for the modern world. Anyone fasting for religious purposes is aiming to feel better about themselves and to feel peace, self-love, and forgiveness. Regardless of your spiritual beliefs, when you are fasting for spiritual purposes, you are doing it to love your body even more and to feel better about yourself.

Physical

Intermittent Fasting plays a major role in healing not only rheumatoid arthritis but also any seizure-related brain damage. More recent studies have shown that IF can reduce the toxic effects of chemotherapy and can also decrease the morbidity rate associated with cancer.

Intermittent Fasting for Better Physical Fitness

When it comes to physical benefits, Intermittent Fasting has an impact on your metabolism, physical endurance, and bodybuilding compatibility.

Better Metabolism

The physical benefits of Intermittent Fasting can be internal or external. Everyone on an Intermittent Fasting program has experienced some internal changes. One of the most important changes is related to the digestive system, as it requires it to consume everything you feed it in a very limited time frame. Therefore, the nutrients you usually consume during a day are now consumed in a very limited time frame. People following an IF program will learn to consume food only when they are hungry during the designated time frame (which is the feeding window), instead of having meals without a specific schedule or choosing mindless eating (eating huge amounts of food, especially junk food).

When you feed your body during a limited time frame, you are also forcing your metabolism to go faster, so your digestive system can process all the food you ate in the feeding window. Also, when you change your diet and go for an LCHF diet, your metabolism becomes a lot more flexible, and it can make it easy for your body to adapt to running on both fats and glucose as energy sources. Therefore, your body becomes like a hybrid organism.

Enhanced Physical Endurance

Intermittent Fasting is usually associated with a lot of physical exercises, as most people who follow this program also indulge in physical activities to maximize the fat-burning process. There is no better way to produce energy than physical exercise, so why not use the energy on working out intensely? Just think of a very important indicator, which is called the "wind" (the volume of oxygen per minute per kilogram of body weight). The higher this indicator is, the higher the physical endurance of the body can get. Obviously, no athlete was able to run that much or that fast right from the beginning. Their endurance improved significantly over time through intense training. Plus, when you burn a lot of fat, your body becomes more agile and strong.

Bodybuilding Compatibility

Intermittent Fasting can work wonders on you if you are a bodybuilder. Now I know this may sound like a paradox, especially when your body is going through nutrient deprivation, but let me explain. The growth hormone can reach unbelievably high levels after 72 hours of fasting, so this is something that bodybuilders should think about. In addition, Intermittent Fasting sets the default fuel type to fats, so your body will burn fats, revealing the muscles below. Bodybuilders are probably used to having 5-6 meals per day, each one having around 2000-2500 calories. In his feeding regimen, they mainly focus on the protein boost, as they are aware that a certain amount of protein is required to maintain their muscle mass. Even though the nutrient intake can be significantly lower, muscle loss during Intermittent Fasting has not been reported (not if you do this process right).

It's said that the recommended amount of protein you need to have per meal is 20 grams, and the total recommended amount per day should be 40 grams. The recommended amount per meal should maximize your muscle growth, but when you are on an Intermittent Fasting program, you may need to have protein supplements to compensate for the amount of protein you need (protein shakes or bars).

Is Intermittent Fasting Safe for Anyone?

IF may have plenty of benefits, so you might think, "What am I waiting for?". Since we are talking about nutrient deprivation, then it's obviously not for everyone. Intermittent Fasting should not be applied to a growing body, so it's definitely not for children or teenagers, at least not for more than 24 hours. You simply shouldn't put a growing body through Intermittent Fasting. As it needs all the nutrients, it can possibly get. Such a procedure is only for fully-grown healthy bodies, and in some cases, it requires the approval of your physician or a nutritionist before you try Intermittent Fasting in order to find out if it's for you.

People might consider that IF doesn't favor women, as they have more delicate bodies, perhaps too delicate for such radical changes. Speaking of women, pregnant women or those breastfeeding their babies should not try Intermittent Fasting. They need all the possible nutrients to feed their unborn or born babies. On top of that, starvation and stress can reduce a woman's fertility, and if you consider those female hunger hormones like leptin and ghrelin are easily triggered when their bodies are underfed, it's a bit more difficult for women to train their mind and digestive system.

However, this shouldn't discourage healthy women from practicing Intermittent Fasting, as if this procedure is done properly, it can lead to increased energy levels and a significant feeling of accomplishment. Women's hormones can be induced by some of the following triggers:

- Not enough sleep, rest or recovery
- Too much stress
- Too much physical exercise
- Infections, inflammation or other illnesses

- Poor food choices or just less food

The aspects mentioned above should not be felt if Intermittent Fasting is done in a proper way. Also, IF shouldn't be tried by people with diabetes who are using insulin. If you are trying to recover from medical interventions or surgeries, you shouldn't be on an Intermittent Fasting program. It goes without saying that people with an eating disorder should not try this procedure. So, if you are experiencing a medical condition, you definitely need to talk to your doctor first before starting IF.

Chapter 5:

Here Is How to Set up a Good Keto Diet

Ketosis and the Ketogenic Diet

Autophagy can be induced by Intermittent Fasting, but also by a keto diet because when you significantly cut down on carbs, you are eliminating the source of glucose from your diet. The Ketogenic Diet is a form of LCHF (low carb high fat) meal plan, in which you are merely replacing carbs with fats. Are you a big fan of processed food, pizza, burgers, bread, pastry, potatoes, or rice? Well, forget about them as this diet will make you rule out these food types from your daily menu. Nutrition plays a vital role when it comes to losing weight; this is why you need to be very careful with the food you are consuming.

The Keto Diet attempts to achieve its namesake, Ketosis, a metabolic state during which plenty of ketones are being released. These chemical compounds are released by your liver and provide energy when the level of glucose is low. Your body can easily adapt to most situations you put it through. Keep in mind that ketosis starts 12 hours after your last meal, and it marks the moment when the body goes into the fat-adapted phase. During this time, your glucose and insulin levels are low enough, while your liver will be releasing ketones which are responsible for providing energy to the cells of your body. At 12 hours since your last meal, your body may not immediately get energy from burning fat, so it runs on ketones instead, as the glucose levels are too low to be used as a valid source of energy.

The whole purpose of the keto diet is to achieve ketosis and also to keep the body in that phase for as long as possible. How can it achieve this? By switching the energy source from glucose to fats. In other words, the ketogenic diet reprograms your body to run on fats instead of glucose from carbs. Now here comes the tricky part! In order to run on fats and to burn fat, you will need to eat fat. This is where the paradox is. How can you get thinner by eating fats? When you think about it, carbs are getting you fat, not necessarily fats. The regular daily diet is rich in carbs, not necessarily in fats. It provides you the excess glucose, which will never be fully consumed by your body. When glucose is not consumed, it goes straight to your blood, raising your blood sugar level, but it also does not release enough energy for you to complete your daily activities.

This means that your body mass will soon turn into fat, as this is made more likely since you are not doing any physical activity at all (or not enough). This may be the solution to the mystery of where body fat comes from. You are increasing your fat tissue on a daily basis unless you are doing something radical to reverse the process. Sure, working out until you "drop" can be one solution, but why not get extra help to burn more fat? Why not switch the default energy source of your body, so it will run on fat instead of glucose. It's like you are a car and you have a tank full of gas, which in this case is fat.

Since your body has only been used to running on glucose, it's really hard for it to recognize any other form of energy source. The problem with carbs is that they cause addiction. This comes from poor quality food, which has little to nothing in terms of nutritional value (it mostly has carbs) but has plenty of calories. These types of food are literally calorie bombs; they are not very consistent; this is why you can get hungry very quickly after that. Very soon, your body will be craving for more carbs. It's a vicious circle that causes a lot of damage to your body and is difficult to escape from.

However, the keto diet could be the solution for you, as it plans to make your body run on an alternative source of energy, which is more "environmentally-friendly." I'm referring, of course, to your body, so if you want to keep it "green," you will need to eat "green." This means more fresh food, more fruits, and more vegetables. During a normal standard diet, you eat carbs like there's no tomorrow. Your diet mainly consists of junk-food and snacks. With the keto diet, you are replacing these carbs with fats (mostly).

Usually, when you hear of fats, you will immediately associate them with toxins. However, there are also healthy fats, saturated fats, which are very good for your body. You will find out more about them during this chapter.

But let's talk about how ketosis starts. When you are suddenly making the switch from glucose to fats, the body will not immediately consume fats, as it's not familiar with them as a source of energy. This is when your liver steps in and releases ketones, chemical compounds that can be used for energy within your body, at least for the moment. Ketones can only be released when the insulin and glucose level are low enough, so the body can't even recognize glucose as a potential source of energy.

We can talk about the benefits of the ketogenic diet for ages, as at the moment it's one of the most popular diets being followed, and for a good reason, as it benefits your health, physical condition, wellbeing, and mood. Somehow, the benefits of the keto diet are intertwined with the ones of Intermittent Fasting and autophagy. Bear in mind that ketosis is just a phase of Intermittent Fasting, and it can induce autophagy.

As you probably know, the keto diet is perhaps the most popular of the LCHF diets, as it delivers outstanding results in terms of health and weight loss. During this diet, you will drop the carbs ratio to a maximum of 15%, or 25% if you want to keep it more moderate, so it's a significant change to your current diet. In order to make such a change, you will need to have basic nutritional knowledge, as you will need the know the food pyramid and the nutritional value for each food type. In other words, you will need to know exactly which foods are your biggest sources of carbs and glucose.

Keto Shopping List

This may sound like a shock to you, but some of the biggest sources of carbs are bread, pastries, potatoes, and rice. Not to mention burgers or pizzas, which are extremely rich in carbs. There is no place in a proper keto diet for any of the food types mentioned above. If you love to snack, bear in mind that chips or sweets will not help you at all in this diet. So, you are probably wondering what exactly you can eat? You will need to make dramatic changes in your refrigerator and throw away every possible processed type of food. You will need to replace them with fresh food, like veggies and fruits, so you will need to shop more often, as these are the most perishable types of foods, and they can spoil easily.

But enough talking, here's what your shopping list will need to contain:

- almonds;
- almond butter;
- beef jerky;
- beef sticks (but be very careful when it comes to checking carbs);
- blackberries;
- Brazil nuts;
- cheese chips;

- cheese slices;
- cheese wedges;
- coconut oil;
- cottage cheese;
- dark chocolate;
- deli meat;
- flaxseed crackers;
- Greek yogurt;
- kale chips;
- sugar-free Jell-O;
- Macadamia nuts;
- Macadamia nut butter;
- olives;
- meat bar;
- peanut butter;
- pecans;
- pepperoni slices;
- pickles;
- pork rinds;
- protein bars (again, be very careful with carb counts);
- pumpkin seeds;
- sardines;
- seaweed snacks;
- smoked oysters;
- sunflower seeds;
- string cheese;
- toasted coconut flakes;
- walnuts;

- avocado;
- cauliflower;
- broccoli;
- eggs;
- mushrooms;
- guacamole;
- peppers;
- and many more.

Now that you've prepared a shopping list for your keto diet, you can look over some keto diet cookbooks to find more recipes on how to cook these ingredients into delicious meals. When you plan to go on a keto diet, you will need to allocate time to shop more often and also to cook almost on a daily basis. You don't have to eat the same food for a few days in a row; you can diversify your menu and come up with your own meal plan in order to eat something different every day of the week.

Now that you have the ingredients and the keto recipes be careful with how you play with the quantities, as you will need to make sure that you will not eat too many calories or too many carbs. The period when you ate huge meals is over. You will now need to eat healthy, with smaller and consistent portions, as this is how you can get into ketosis. Eating massive amounts of food will not get you into ketosis, so you will need to train your body to have lower portions of food that are better balanced, with a maximum 15% carbs ratio.

You might want to add to your shopping list, fish, fish oil (as it's rich in omega 3), and of course, olive oil. Are you wondering about which kind of fats are healthy for your body? Well, here they are! Omega 3 fats from fish or olive oil are just a few examples of healthy fats. Fruits and veggies should not be missing from your keto diet, but you can also add in some pork, beef, or chicken once in a while. Be very careful with the quantities, as they are also sources of glucose, so you don't want to eat too much of them. I know this will sound a bit too difficult, but you will need to portion your food properly, so you will need to put the exact quantity on your plate and not 100 grams more.

To sum up, the keto diet should be based on the following ingredients:

- fruits;
- vegetables;
- dairy products (cheese, yogurt);
- seeds;
- healthy fat oils; and
- fish and meat (in lower quantity).

When it comes to keto drinks, you can mostly rely on water to never let you down, but you can also consume coffee or herbal/green tea (no sugar, though).

Benefits of Ketosis and the Ketogenic Diet

There are plenty of positive facts about ketosis, ketones, and the keto diet, but have you ever wondered what exactly the benefits of this metabolic state and meal plan are? Well, let's start with ketosis first. Some of the main advantages and benefits of this state are:

1) More control over your appetite. Ketosis is the first state of Intermittent Fasting, a transition period which marks the end of using glucose as an energy source and switching over to your fat reserves. Plenty of people who were in this state have confirmed that they felt a lot less hunger than expected (remember, you are 12 hours away from your last meal). Studies confirm the loss of appetite in this phase, so it's a lot different from the period when your body was hooked on carbs, which represent the main source of glucose. The keto diet is designed to (almost completely) eliminate carbs and glucose

from your daily meals, thus preventing the rise of insulin and blood sugar levels.

2) Potential weight loss. We have to acknowledge that proteins and fats are the most useful macronutrients, and in order to activate the state of ketosis, the body has to become fat-adapted. This means significantly cutting down on carbs or eliminating them, just to prevent any consumption of glucose. When you feed your body fats, it will burn fats, so they become the primary energy source for your body. The role of ketones is to extract the energy from your fat tissue, so they are the tools the body uses to break down the fat tissue. The more you extend ketosis, the more fat you can burn. As mentioned above, the state of ketosis suppresses your appetite, so you will no longer crave carbs or glucose. This will lead to a lower insulin level and blood sugar, all while the amount of ketones is growing at a very fast pace, and this can only favor the fat burning process (leading to more fat/weight loss).

3) Prediabetes and diabetes reversal. A funny fact about insulin is that it needs to be at a very low level to regulate blood sugar. When your body is constantly consuming glucose, then you can only increase the insulin level and also the blood sugar level. When you stop feeding

glucose to your body, this will allow the insulin level to decrease until it will eventually do its job and regulate the level of glucose in your blood. Ketosis is what encourages lower levels of insulin, as this state of glucose deprivation enhances the insulin's function. Those two indicators are what you need to look after when you are in a prediabetes or diabetes phase. When they are extremely high, there are high chances that you could be suffering from one of these conditions or diseases. However, lower levels of these indicators will reverse these conditions, until people can claim they are "cured" of prediabetes or diabetes.

4) Better athletic performance. The fat burning process can melt down your fat reserves, but it can also enhance your muscle mass at the same time. More muscles and less fat can only lead to a stronger, more agile, and faster body, so in other words, it can lead to better athletic performance.

5) Epilepsy control. As it turns out, the keto diet can prove to be extremely efficient in controlling epilepsy for adults or children, even when the subjects didn't respond too well to anti-seizure medication.

Chapter 6:

Let's Talk About Intermittent Fasting, but What Should We Drink? Here Are the Best Drinks

Hydration plays a very important role in Intermittent Fasting; this is why we all need to hydrate properly when following such a program. For a normal person, there are some requirements saying that we need to consume at least 2 liters of water (or liquids) per day. But how many of us are really sticking to this rule? I personally know people that have completely replaced water with other drinks. They are drinking teas, coffees, and plenty of sodas. However, what's the total amount of sugar you are consuming per day? Have you looked over a can of Coca-Cola to see how much sugar it has? Even when you have the diet version, it's still not healthy enough.

Truth be told, water is the complete drink you can think of. It's the perfect "cure" for your thirst, it can refresh you, and can even have a minor quantity of vitamins and minerals. Water can help you with metabolism and detox, and possibly the best part of all; it doesn't have any calories. This is why water is used by people during Intermittent Fasting. If you are feeling thirsty, obviously, you will need to stay away from soft drinks and stick to water. It should help your organs function at an optimal level; this is why you need to drink a lot of it and refill frequently. With Intermittent Fasting, you may need to drink more water than when you are on your standard meal plan. The water requirement may be influenced by the weight of your body, the more you weigh, the more water you need to drink. Still, it's recommended to drink water every 30 to 50 minutes, not just when you are thirsty. So far, water has proven to be a great hunger suppressor, as when you drink it, you tend not to feel hungry anymore. It tricks your brain and your stomach, and it gives them a satisfying sensation, at least for a while.

There are plenty of advantages associated with drinking water, most of them are mentioned above, but if you want to drink higher quality water, or possibly alkaline water, you will need to get bottled water, as tap water may have a higher concentration of chlorine and this is definitely not good for your body and internal organs. This is why you will need to drink something else also, not just water, something like a secondary drink which you do not have as often as water. Some good alternatives would be tea, coffee, or apple cider vinegar, but they all have to be sugar-free.

You are probably in love with sugar, you can hardly picture your life without it, but eliminating sugar from your food and drinks is mandatory in order to have a healthy life. Sugar can be considered responsible for more deaths than all the other dangerous substances put together (alcohol, drugs, tobacco, and so on). Do you know that a simple can of Coca-Cola has around 40% sugar? Now that's a huge concentration, a lethal dose if you'd like, especially if you drink it on a regular basis. You will probably think again when buying this drink for your kids or for yourself.

You can have other drinks as well, with much less sugar, or possibly, no sugar at all. Keep in mind that sugar literally means glucose, and it's something you need to avoid consuming when you are following this program. If you are thinking of replacing soft drinks with fresh-squeezed orange juice, or other types of juices, bear in mind that they also have a very high concentration of sugar. Just to make things easier, you need to avoid any sweet drink. If you feel like drinking tea, don't put any sugar in it. You might want to stay away from honey as well, even though it has excellent effects on your health, it still contains glucose.

Some specialists would recommend completely eliminating any fruit drinks, including fruit tea, especially any type of tea made from berries (they are very sweet to start with). Now it's up to you if you want to be that radical, but sweet means glucose (even though it doesn't come from sugar), and you need to avoid or to limit your glucose intake during this program seriously. The sweetness of the drink is always something you need to consider, but what about the vitality it can bring to you?

When it comes to energy and vitality in a drink, nothing beats caffeine. This is why drinking coffee or black tea is highly recommended when you are following this program. This doesn't mean that you have to become a coffee addict. Almost every adult person on this planet drinks coffee, so why shouldn't you? Coffee seems like part of our life, something that we can't live without. In this case, you shouldn't drink more than 2-4 cups of coffee per day, as this quantity should be more than enough to provide you the energy you need for the whole day. Energy can make you burn more fat; burning fat will release more energy. It's a cycle that shouldn't stop, and if you are giving caffeine to your body, you are preventing this cycle from stopping.

Coffee is known to increase your blood pressure, so if you have any health conditions that affect your blood pressure, you shouldn't drink too much coffee, as you don't want your blood pressure to skyrocket. If you are an agitated person by nature, then you will need to keep your coffee consumption as low as possible. If you are a calmer person, then you can drink more coffee, as long as you respect the daily recommended dosage.

Coffee can give you energy and vitality but also plays a very important role in your metabolism. So, yes, the myth is true! Coffee does make you go to the bathroom. Since it has that effect on you, it's also highly recommended in detox, as it helps your body to cleanse from all the stored toxins. However, these toxins are protected by fat tissue, so this can only mean that, since coffee facilitates burning fat, it lets those toxins free and eliminates them before they affect your internal organs.

Now that you realize the importance of coffee, you are probably thinking of heading over to your nearest supermarket and buying more coffee. However, as we all know, pure coffee doesn't have the best taste, does it? It's so bitter that you often want to sweeten it. This is mistake number one! No matter how bitter coffee is, you still need to avoid any sugar (even if it's brown sugar) or honey. If you really can't stand the taste of coffee but feel like you want to drink it, then you will need to use stevia for sweetening.

If you are a hardcore coffee drinker, then the taste of the coffee will not make you sweeten it. You can have the strongest coffee without putting any sweetener in it, natural or artificial, and without putting anything else, so no cream, milk (soy, almond, skimmed, semi-skimmed, whole, or foam milk), not even cinnamon. There are plenty of things and spices you can put in a coffee, but a hardcore coffee drinker will not bother with any of them. His specialty is the bulletproof coffee, as this is a coffee beverage made with high-quality coffee beans and high-quality fats. This is how you can avoid consuming any glucose with a simple coffee.

However, if you are not a hardcore coffee drinker, this doesn't mean that you shouldn't have this drink just because you can't drink it "bulletproof." Coffee shops all over the world have created art around coffee making, but they add so much stuff to your coffee that coffee may not be the best choice for you, especially if you are on an Intermittent Fasting program.

You don't have to be a "purist" to have a coffee, so you can "spoil" your coffee with some add-ons or spices. Still, you will need to keep an eye on the calories as well, so you really can't put that much cream or milk. If you really have to use milk, you can use almond or soy milk. They are both tasty enough to go with your coffee, and they have fewer calories and a minimum amount of carbs. As a sweetener, I would highly recommend stevia, perhaps the healthiest and best choice when it comes to sweetening a drink. If you can't have stevia, then you can go ahead with brown sugar, which is a less dangerous form of sugar (honey is way too sweet in this case and may have higher levels of glucose).

Adding some cinnamon to your coffee can be an innocent way to add some flavor to your drink, and it shouldn't affect the calorie or glucose intake. When preparing your coffee, it's highly recommended not to add all of these add-ons in your coffee. Just add one or at a maximum of two. Personally, If I were to choose from these three, I would go with almond milk and cinnamon, so no sweetener at all. However, this is your call. During this program, you may also need to watch the calorie and glucose intake, so it's up to you how you play with the quantities in your coffee.

If you must drink tea without sweetening it, so without any sugar or honey (not even fruit tea), coffee obviously has to be as bitter as possible to be more effective for your fat loss process. You can also try some apple cider vinegar during Intermittent Fasting. However, I would strongly advise moderate quantities for this drink.

All of these alternatives should not replace water as your main drink of the day. You can have between 2-4 cups of coffee per day, and let's say about the same number of cups of tea per day. But you will still need to drink mainly water, as this is the drink that helps your internal organs the most. All of the other drinks already contain water, so you are just consuming water in different forms or flavors. Proper hydration will help you with your metabolism, self-cleansing process (detox), and with the proper function of your organs. It can give you the energy and vitality you need for the rest of the day in order to continue your fat burning process at optimal levels.

Chapter 7:

How to Live a Healthy Life Thanks to the Constancy of Physical Exercise

Let's just admit it! Most of us are very lazy when it comes to physical activity; we live a very passive lifestyle. We are so caught up in the daily stress, daily tasks from our job, and commuting that we barely have time to engage in any physical activity. Your app on your phone shows that you are far from the daily 10,000 steps recommended for a healthy lifestyle. When you are always in a hurry to get your kids to school or to get to work on time, take care of all the daily tasks, have a quick lunch, and drive back home, it's very hard to imagine yourself doing any sort of physical activity. On top of that, there are plenty of us who have a part-time job, so we are working at least 12 hours per day, and if you add the hours spent in traffic, it's really hard to imagine having any time or energy for physical exercise.

This is the most common excuse we like to tell ourselves when it comes to working out. However, if we can allocate ourselves enough time for these kinds of activities, we will soon discover its benefits. Now, I know what you are thinking: "I barely have time or energy; it's literally impossible to spend some time working out." Remember, energy is released when working out, so if you just think of this aspect, then you will find extra motivation to work out. Therefore, not only you will feel energized, but you will also look and feel great. Some people have already understood the importance of physical activity and apply this knowledge in their life. You can see people using the bike to go to work; some gyms are pretty crowded at 6 - 7 AM, you even see people swimming pools or jogging early in the morning.

People are not ashamed to work out in the morning before going to work. They can have an intense workout, followed by a quick shower, and then head to work. There is no better way to get in a positive mood, to feel great, and to have vitality for the whole day. Forget about any pills you are taking to have vitality or energy, the solution is available for anyone, and it's called physical exercise (although some vitamins won't do you any harm if you take them when you start your day).

In this chapter, we will cover some of the most basic forms of physical exercise you can practice daily. When you combine this type of activity with Intermittent Fasting, it's always better to practice it during the first hours of your day, even before you had your first meal (IF may involve skipping breakfast, as you are about to see in the next chapter of this book). The answer is very simple. The chances are that you are already at least 12 hours from your last meal, and your body is in the fat-adapted phase. Therefore, when you apply physical stress (workout) on your body, the fat tissue will be used for energy. Burning your fat reserves will release the energy stored in there, and guess what? You will lose fat. This is why working out in the morning on an empty stomach is the best way to lose weight/fat. Plus, it can give you the energy you need for the rest of the day.

Jogging

A very popular type of physical activity is jogging. It's free, it's effective, but it requires physical endurance, even so, it's really not that hard. Have you ever seen any athlete or marathon runner who is overweight? I know I haven't. This is why these guys run a lot. They run plenty of miles every day, and it's working wonders for them. If you practice jogging, you will have your cardio function at its best. Some people prefer to run on the streets, others on the treadmill at the gym. Personally, I recommend outdoor running, as you can easily adjust your pace. You won't be working out just your leg muscles either, as you will notice how much fat you will burn from your abs.

Experts came to recommend walking at least 10,000 steps each day. This is the daily recommended "dosage" for a healthy person. You will be burning a few hundred calories if you walk that much. The good news with jogging is that you will be burning a lot more calories if you run for that distance. This equates to approximately 5 miles of running. If you aren't training for a marathon, then this should be plenty for you, but if you are training for one, then you will need to run a lot more. Most physicians recommend at least 30 minutes of physical exercise each day but imagine the results you can have if you jog uninterrupted for 30 minutes. It can be one of the most effective types of exercise you can practice.

Obviously, running just 1 mile will not be sufficient unless you are a beginner when it comes to jogging. You need to make running a habit, so you might want to have a gym membership (if it has treadmills) for those times when the weather outside is not quite jogging-friendly. We would all like California's weather, but if you are reading this from other parts of the world, then perhaps the weather out there is more rainy and windy than sunny and warm.

Even if you start with just 1 mile of running, you will need to increase the distance you run for constantly. In the beginning, 5 miles will probably sound like an impossible distance to run, but don't worry; you will get there in time! Also, you will notice how good you will feel how much weight you have lost, and perhaps you will need to change your clothes as you will need smaller sizes. Not too bad!

Resistance Training

When you want to have increased ability, to be more of an athlete than an amateur, then you will need to spend a lot more time training. You might want to train yourself for a competition, like a marathon or perhaps the "Ironman triathlon." Then you will need to spend a lot of time running, riding your bike and swimming. In this case, 30 minutes of jogging will simply not be enough. You are at a totally different level, and this time, you are not working out to lose fat or weight, you are building resistance and muscle mass.

If you want to run the New York City Marathon or any other marathon, then you will need to run a lot, as 5 miles will definitely not be enough. You will need to know how to dose your effort, how to master breathing (getting oxygen to your lungs and muscles is crucial), or how to hydrate yourself properly. Soccer players are able to run for 90 minutes at a very intense pace, and they can cover 8-9 miles during a game. Most men (that participate in this competition) can run a marathon within 3 hours and 30 minutes to 4 hours. The record is a little more than 2 hours. To run 26.2 miles in a bit more than 2 hours is absolutely amazing. If you have serious traffic, you might spend more time driving than this man who set the record for a marathon run.

There isn't a more difficult competition than the "Ironman triathlon." If you feel like the ultimate athlete, then you could test yourself in such a competition. It involves a 2.4-mile swim, a 112-mile bicycle ride, and a 26.2-mile marathon, in this order. It's an amazing performance to finish such a race, and even race in it is something out of this world. Obviously, such a competition is for elite athletes, so you will need to have outstanding physical endurance.

When it comes to any form of resistance training or exercises, you will need to have ambition beyond imagination. Nothing should stand in your way as you will have to keep going and not stop until you have reached your goals. Of course, it's also about how you feel, as you can't push yourself too hard if you don't feel that you are up to it. You don't have to give yourself a heart attack just because you had to keep going no matter what. Pushing your limits should be done in a very responsible way; you shouldn't endanger your health.

Swimming

If you have access to a swimming pool and if you can swim, then this activity is a must for you. If you don't know how to swim, then you will need to learn, as this is one of the best and most enjoyable workouts out there. It's hard to think of any physical activity that involves most of the muscles of your body. Well, this is what swimming is about. It involves your legs muscles, arm muscles, chest, back, abs, all major groups are exercised during swimming.

This means that wherever you have fat stored, it will be burned as this practice applies "pressure" to all areas of your body. This is why all professional swimmers have lean bodies.

If you plan to participate in a sports activity, swimming is highly recommended, as it's a very pleasant and easy way to burn fat and work on most muscles throughout your body. Just like in every physical exercise, breathing plays a crucial role. It can make the whole difference between being exhausted and about to sink and to swim without any problems for a long distance. Although I haven't covered this for other forms of physical activities, before you start swimming (just like any other form of training or workout), you need to prepare your body, especially your muscles. You need to warm up, get some blood to these muscles, as you don't want to experience muscle cramps when you are in the middle of a lake. True swimmers know how to handle these situations, and to get over those cramps and eventually continue swimming. However, if you properly warm-up before swimming, you will not have difficulties during your swim — this why such a practice is mandatory before diving in the swimming pool, lake, or sea.

Playing Sports

Who said you only need to engage in physical activities just during mornings? You can spend a lot of quality time with your friends playing sports. This can be a more moderate type of physical activity, but why not burn some calories and have some fun while you're doing it? You don't have to meet up with the guys just to have a couple of drinks. You can also join them and play basketball, football, baseball, tennis, squash, or soccer. It's not written anywhere that you have to be a professional player to practice these sports. Being a fan is more than cheering for your favorite team in the stands; you can also practice the sport and better understand it.

Therefore, meet your friends in the park or at a playground and practice your favorite sport over there. You will not run as much as the players from your favorite team, but you will burn some extra calories in the afternoons or evenings when you usually have very consistent meals. This is one healthy way to spend your free time.

Working Out at the Gym

If you fancy a more static activity, then you will need to head over to the gym. It will allow you to work on every muscle group you have, so you will not be ignoring any particular one. Gyms are very popular nowadays, especially if they allow you to practice all kinds of activities like fitness, aerobics, pilates, or other activities for ladies, bodybuilding, treadmills, cardio, TRX, and other activities for men. There are plenty of gyms that also have swimming pools and saunas to provide a complete experience. Therefore, you can find everything you need in one place.

When you combine working out with Intermittent Fasting, it's always better to head to the gym in the morning and exercise on an empty stomach (you already know why). This has to become a habit, so you need to create your own workout plan, divided by days. Since you are lifting weights, it's crucial to exercise correctly, as you don't want to hurt yourself or to do any damage to your spine. There are many amateurs who don't work out correctly, as they always want to try heavy lifting since they somehow feel that the gym is about getting more physical strength.

There is no shame in working out with light weights, you can learn how to exercise correctly, plus you can have plenty of repetitions, and this can be a very good strategy if you plan to burn fat. Breathing can make a huge difference, as it can give you the strength to lift all these weights. You can maximize the efficiency of weight lifting by taking a lung full of oxygen every time you lift.

HIIT (High-Intensity Interval Training)

If you are planning to use this method of training, then you definitely mean business. As it turns out, HIIT is one of the most effective methods of training, as proven by research conducted by Dr. Izumi Tabata. The study was conducted in 1996 over a period of 6 weeks. It was tracking the VO2 max level, which is the rate of oxygen consumption during physical training. The participants were divided into two groups:

- The members of the control group who were allowed to train 60 minutes per day (moderate-intensity training), five times per week. The study results showed that they reached just 70% VO2 max. This type

of practice is also known as low-intensity steady-state cardio or LISS.
- The members of the other group had a different approach called HIIT (High-Intensity Interval Training), having very intense sessions of training at 170% VO2 max. They were having 20/10 sessions, which means they had 20 seconds of extremely intense workout, they would have a break for 10 seconds and then repeat the same procedure again. They repeated the whole process eight times, so in 4 minutes, they had very intense exercise with eight rounds of training and pause.

After six weeks, the results were staggering. The control group had about 1800 minutes of training, compared to just 120 minutes of training for the HIIT group. For the LISS group, the VO2 max increased from 53 +/- 5 ml kg^{-1} min^{-1} to 58 +/- 3 ml kg^{-1} min^{-1}, but there wasn't too much difference in their anaerobic capacity. In the meantime, the HIIT group had outstanding results. Their VO2 max levels increased by 7ml. kg^{-1} min^{-1}, while their anaerobic capacity was enhanced by 28%.

In addition, the study showed that the people practicing HIIT were more effective when it comes to physiological adaptations, plus it's also more time-efficient than LISS. If you are looking for an answer, it's very simple. When you apply the weight stress factor, your body is way more responsive. You can also try it at the gym, and you will notice that you will have way better results if you lift very heavy weights just a few times than if you lift light weights too many times.

The study also discovered:

a) The VO2 max levels significantly improved for the LISS group. The body of the people involved in this group got more efficient when it was working out at lower intensities, so they are able to try more intense training. Their bodies were becoming fitter as they were used to working at lower intensities.

b) In the case of HIIT members, their VO2 max improved a lot, even though it started at a lower level. There is always room to improve. The members of the LISS group were already fitter, and it was extremely difficult to notice any kind of improvement.

c) The VO2 max level was still lower at the end of the study for the people in the HIIT group, compared to the ones from the LISS group. Those from the HIIT group didn't become a lot fitter, but still, their relative fitness enhanced more.

If you are a bit confused, just look at the overall results. The HIIT group enhanced their aerobic and anaerobic fitness, and you simply can't say the same thing about the LISS group. And this was all achieved through 4 minutes of training a day. Just imagine the results of longer training. Obviously, unless you are looking to improve your endurance, there is really no point in doing cardio at your gym for a very long time. If you are simply aiming to become healthier and fitter, then high-intensity interval training proved to be a lot more efficient method of exercise than regular gym training at a lower intensity. As it turns out, the HIIT method not only saves you plenty of time, but it also helps you preserve your joints and can lead to better metabolism.

This type of training is known for increasing the capability of mitochondria to produce energy, with a 69% improvement in senior people and 49% in younger adults. You can't expect to train in HIIT mode for 75 minutes straight like you would do with a low-intensity workout, but just imagine what the results of a longer HIIT practice would be. When you train for about 30 minutes this way, it will have serious autophagic effects. Bear in mind that muscles are stimulated a lot better through high-intensity workouts, so don't worry about muscle loss, as the more weight you apply to your workout, the more you will be stimulating your muscle growth. If you want to avoid sarcopenia (loss of skeletal muscles) or just muscle waste, then combining HIIT with endurance training is one of the best methods. You will soon see how your muscles will start growing while your fat tissue starts decreasing.

Muscular Soreness

Among the weird reasons why people avoid having an active lifestyle and doing physical exercises is muscle soreness (besides getting sweaty). People are thinking: "Why should I cause this pain to myself?". Developing your muscles should be considered a must. Now, of course, you don't have to build your muscles like Arnold Schwarzenegger, but you still need to build your muscles to protect your health and mobility. So why not have some muscles instead of some fat? You will feel and look great! You don't need better motivation than this.

If you want to look better and replace fat with muscles, working out is mandatory. Don't believe that there are types of food that will just melt the fat away from you while you do nothing instead. Unfortunately, muscles can only be built the hard way. Therefore, it requires hard work and dedication, and it also involves some pain. Yep! No pain, no gain! This is the motto of every bodybuilder! If you truly want to look great, to have a body others will envy, then you need to commit to serious high-intensity training. As you are trying to reach a higher level, your muscles will not be used to so much stress (which comes out of many repetitions, heavier weights, or longer distances ran). Don't worry, this is just the response of your muscles when you are transitioning into a different phase, and it can be considered a sign of muscle growth. Therefore, I like to consider muscle soreness "a sign of being alive."

Muscle soreness may last for a longer period of time, but it's important that you don't stop training just because you are in this condition. You are not handicapped, so you shouldn't stop. In fact, if you keep going, you will notice the pain goes away, so the best way to get rid of it is to keep going. A massage over the zone will be fine, but the muscles have to move in order to make the pain go away. This is far more effective than sitting around and waiting for the pain to go away.

Daily Exercise

Physical exercise should be done on a daily basis; this is how we can stay healthy and look a lot better, plus have vitality like never before. I believe at least 30 minutes of daily exercise should be done, regardless of whether you are jogging, working out or swimming. This will lead to at least 150 minutes per week (assuming that you like to keep your weekends relaxing). If you don't feel like going to the gym, doing some push-ups and sit-ups will always do you good, but it's highly recommended to try jogging as well, or swimming, if you know how to swim and have access to a swimming pool.

I like to think of this way of exercising as a maintenance workout. When you are just doing some minor exercises at home, but you don't combine them with anything else, like jogging or swimming. This will not give you spectacular results. You will maintain your muscle mass, but you will not be burning too much fat. Fat burning usually happens when you switch to jogging or swimming, as the intensity is a bit higher.

If you do want to lose more weight and to look great, 30 minutes per day will simply not be enough. You will need to train for at least 75 minutes per day, or a total of at least 450 minutes per week. Obviously, the intensity of your training can determine how much fat you will be burning. Keep in mind that your training session should not be kept at the same level of intensity forever. As you train more, you will need to add more intensity to your training, as this is the only way you can progress. You will need to push your limits if you want to achieve more. Obviously, it's not necessary to become an "Iron man" athlete, but if you want to look great, be healthy and improve your physical endurance, then you will need to train more and harder over time.

Chapter 8:

Let Us Immediately Set a New Mentality

Intermittent Fasting is more than a weight loss program; it's a lifestyle with plenty of benefits to your health. When we are living in these modern times, and we eat so much processed and unhealthy food IF can help us train our body to be more efficient and self-protective by bringing some discipline to our daily meal schedule. It can help us divide the day into a feeding window and a fasting period, but we need to avoid confusion as the feeding window is not quite the same thing as the fed state, and the fasting period may not mean the same thing as the fast state.

Therefore, you will need first to understand the different phases of Intermittent Fasting:

- When it's been 12 hours since your last meal, your body enters the fast state as well as the metabolic state of ketosis (which has something to do with the keto diet). It's within this period when the

body uses fat cells for energy, so it switches the primary energy source from glucose to fats. Therefore, this is when your body starts to burn fat (or to run on fats).
- After 18 hours of fasting, the body enters the fat-burning mode. During this phase, the body is generating huge amounts of ketones, and blood ketones levels are a lot higher than in normal conditions.
- After 24 hours of fasting, your body enters the autophagy phase, when old cells or misfolded proteins associated with Alzheimer's disease or other illnesses are being recycled or replaced.
- Surprisingly, after 48 hours since your last meal, growth hormone levels skyrocket, as it now has a level 5 times higher than the one at the beginning of the fasting period. This is shocking, as you are no longer feeding your body, and the lack of calories, carbs, or proteins can lead to this situation. (This can be a very useful tip for bodybuilders.)
- When it has been at least 54 hours since your last meal, insulin levels reach their lowest point of the fast period, and this can only mean that your body is becoming a lot more insulin-sensitive.

- When it has been 72 hours since your last meal, your body is destroying old immune cells and develops new ones.

Intermittent Fasting is more about planning your meals than what you eat, although eating healthy is highly recommended with this procedure. Unless you are experiencing some medical condition, you should definitely try IF and choose from one of its programs:

- The Leangains Program
- The Warrior Diet
- Eat Stop Eat Diet
- The Alternate-Day Fast
- Water Fast

So, let's detail them one by one to find out more details about them.

The Leangains Program or the 16/8 Hours Fast

This method is one of the most popular fast procedures, and as you probably noticed, it's pretty self-explanatory because it divides the day into a 16 hour fasting period and an 8-hour feeding window. It's important to note the difference between the fasting period and the fast state. The fasting period refers to the period you are not eating at all, while the fast state refers to the period when the body runs on fats after glucose is no longer available. The fasting period can start immediately after your last meal, while the fast state will not start until 12 hours after you had your last meal.

This program is also known as the Leangains method, and it's one of the few daily fasting methods. Applying this procedure on a daily basis can have amazing results for the fat burning process, as 16 hours of fasting should be more than enough to burn some of your fat reserves. There are 4 hours of fast state, so it's important to do something during this period to maximize the fat loss process. If you follow the rules below, you might have better results with this method:

- Protein boosts are needed with most meals (whenever possible).
- Working out is highly recommended, so any form of physical exercise should be linked to this program, as fasting will work better.
- If you are still a carb addict, then you will need to consume them on your training days, as you don't want glucose getting to your blood if it's not consumed. When

you are not training, try to cut down on carbs as much as possible.
- During your feeding period, you can enjoy consistent meals (although you don't have to overeat just to compensate for the whole day within these 8 hours). Are you used to snacking? Forget about it, especially during your fasting period, when you should only drink water (preferably).
- Your first meal of the day should be the most consistent one, regardless of whether you are working out or not on that specific day.
- It's highly unlikely for this method to lead to muscle loss (16 hours of fasting during a day should not cause this issue), but if you are concerned about this issue, you can take BCAA (branched-chain amino acids), just to avoid any possible muscle loss during training in the fasting period.

If you are planning to use this method, then you will need to consider all of the following:

1) Set when you start your fasting period, so you need to plan accordingly because you will have 16 hours without calorie intake. This is why it's highly recommended to start your fasting period

in the evenings. You can have your last meal at 6 PM (or if you prefer at 8 PM), so you can have the next meal at 10 AM (or noon, for the second situation). Guess what? After you entered the fast state, that's when it's the best time to work out. So you can start after 6 AM or after 8 AM, depending on when you had your last meal.

2) After setting your fasting period, you will be "stuck" with the feeding period. If you go for the 6 PM to 10 AM fasting period, then you will need to eat between 10 AM and 6 PM, not outside this window. The more you get used to fasting, the more you should be able to increase your fasting period and reduce the feeding one. This is why the Leangains Program can have an 18 hour fasting period.

3) You will need to decide when it's the best time to train. This depends a lot on the time of your last meal, but if you had dinner and nothing else to eat afterward, then you can start your training at 6-7 AM in the morning. It's up to you how long you want to train, as you are probably in a hurry to get to work. However, even if you are training at a moderate intensity, you should still limit your workout to 75 minutes (that's plenty of time for you).

4) Although there are no specific requirements, it's also important to eat proper food during

your feeding window. If your definition of food is returning to fast-food (burgers, pizza, French fries, and so on), then you need to reinvent your daily menu completely. Try something healthy instead! Something a lot lower in carbs and a lot more nutritious. Following a keto diet seems to be the best choice when being on an Intermittent Fasting Program.

The Warrior Diet

Developed by Ori Hofmekler, this plan is inspired by the lifestyle of Spartan warriors from Ancient Greece. It's a different approach to daily fasting, and a lot more radical than the Leangains program as it involves 20 hours of uninterrupted fasting. This means that you will only have four hours per day to eat. Now you can imagine that in Ancient Greece, in times of war, the Spartan warrior didn't have time for three meals per day. He only had time for one meal per day (a massive meal), so this eating habit inspired the warrior diet.

When your feeding window is limited to just 4 hours, you simply can't have two full meals during this period. This is why you will need a complete meal, filled with every possible macronutrient your body needs. Of course, you don't have to be at war to experience this diet; in fact, you can try it anytime, as it has plenty of benefits for your body. It's highly recommended to consume only water during the fasting period; however, when you are starting this diet, and you are not used to it, you can also try some fruit instead of sugary snacks (chips or sweets are totally forbidden in such a program).

The rule is simple. The more you fast, the more fat you will burn. Just think about it! The body has 8 hours in the fast state, that's the time to act, that's the time to train. Indeed, this plan can work wonders if you train intensively in a fast state. It's highly recommended that you stick to this plan if you have fat to burn because as long as there is fat to burn, you don't have to worry about any muscle loss. If you are planning to follow this program, then there are some rules you will need to follow:

- Stick to the 20 hours fasting period on a daily basis. (You can lower it to 18 hours if you think 20 hours is too much, but you still need to stick to it.)
- Snacks have to be replaced, so it's OK to have some fruits or veggies instead, mostly in the feeding period. If you think that 18-20 hours is too much without having anything to eat, then you can try a

fruit or veggie (moderate quantities) during the fasting period.
- Make sure your meal is consistent enough, as you will need to cover the protein requirements for the whole day with that meal. Proteins are required to maintain muscle mass, so it's very important that you consider this when cooking your meal. It all depends on the amount of muscle you already have, but the general rule of thumb is that it should be 1 gram of protein for every pound of body weight.
- This program may involve counting calories, so it's highly important to make sure you have the necessary calorie intake for the whole day. The meal will have to be consistent enough and will also need to have high nutrient value.

Here are some basic instructions that you will need to apply for this Intermittent Fasting program:

- Your feeding window is only 4 hours long (6 maximum), so you will need to decide when you will want to set it, whether it's at breakfast, lunch, or dinner.
- The duration of your feeding period should be between 4 and 6 hours.

- It's your call if you want to have a snack during the fasting period. Keep in mind that chips or sweets should be avoided at all costs. If you really want to have some snacks during that period, you will need to stick to fruit or vegetables. Protein shakes are highly recommended during this period if you really feel the need to have something. If you feel up to it, then you can keep your fasting period "pure."

Speaking of no-nos if you want to follow this program, here's what you need to avoid:

- Obviously, chips and sweets are forbidden. You will need to stay away from pastries as well, as they're a great source of carbs. Any type of food that is rich in carbs should be avoided in this program. Potatoes, rice, bread, pasta, pizza, burgers, pastries, sweets, soft drinks, and so on are great sources of carbs and sugar. If you are on such a program, you will need to exclude them from your daily menu (or significantly cut down on them).
- The fasting period should be kept for fasting, not for eating anything (besides some low-calorie snacks composed of fruits and veggies).

- When you set the time of your feeding window, you will have to keep it at the same time every day. You should not have your meal at dinner time one day, and at noon, or even earlier the next day.

Based on the facts presented above, the fasting period is known as the undereating period in this program, whilst the feeding window is the overeating period. The Warrior Diet is probably not something you want to keep for a very long time; this is why it's structured in three different weeks. During the first week of this program, you will focus more on detox. The second week is all about consuming high fats, and in the last week, you will be focusing on the fat loss process. There are even detailed menus for The Warrior Diet, which are compliant with the "theme" of the week.

Here are some principles you will need to stick to when following this program:

1) Don't hesitate to use more fat! The fat burning process happens in the mitochondria. This process unites inner cells that use energy. There are plenty of mitochondrial enzymes being released, so there are higher chances for a successful fat burning process. Just think of the mitochondria as an interesting collection of tissues, and the muscle mass represents the

biggest collection of all. It's thought that a certain type of muscle can determine fat usage.

2) Enhance your energy turnover. Bear in mind that more energy means more fat burn. These two aspects are intertwined. If you want to release more energy, you will need to burn fat. If you want to burn fat, you will need to release more energy. Makes sense, right? When your body is in a fasted state, the only source of energy can come from your fat reserves. Your body is not like a hybrid car, which runs on petrol and electric power as well. In this case, you only have one source of energy, the fat reserves. However, maintaining a very high level of energy can be very difficult when you are eating only during the feeding window. This is why some specialists would recommend having a minor snack to boost your energy during the fasting period. Minerals and vitamins are what you need, and you can get them from fruits and veggies. Make sure you avoid glucose, as this will stop your fasted state. Also, it's highly recommended to drink water and coffee.

3) Improve the detox process. Many people see Intermittent Fasting as a great way to promote self-cleansing and detox. It stimulates your metabolism, so in order to make it work

properly, you will need to consume food rich in antioxidants (fruits and veggies).

Nothing is for sure in this world, and the principles above can't guarantee the success of your Warrior Diet, but they can surely increase the chances of success. If you are experiencing poor results with the fat loss process or simply not getting the results you expect, perhaps you might want to take a look below:

- Your body may be insulin resistant. When it's already used with loads of glucose coming from carbs, then your body will not react as you might expect, and the glucose or insulin level will simply not decrease. You trained your body only to work on glucose, so it can't even consider a different source of energy (like the fat tissue). Your body will be craving carbs, and as long as it has a high glucose level, it can only run on this source of energy and not on fat reserves.
- You probably have higher than usual levels of toxins. Toxins and fats can be linked together, so whenever you have higher toxins levels, the chances are that you are also fatter. In this case, the fat tissue plays a role in protecting the toxins. Instead of being released,

cleansed out of your body, these toxins will be affecting your internal organs. Intermittent Fasting can give you a hand with releasing those toxins, but the consumption of fruits and vegetables (with a higher concentration of antioxidants) will also help you. Bear in mind that detox can be activated by fasting or undereating between 10 and 18 hours. Constipation may be blocking the detox process, but you can avoid it if you consume fruits, veggies, and food rich in fiber.

- Fluctuating estrogen can block the fat loss process for women. In this case, the fat tissue may act as an estrogen regulator, as it's releasing aromatase enzymes, which can turn testosterone into estrogen. Therefore, the estrogen level is being regulated, and this means that ladies will not have to deal with reduced bone density, messing up the menstrual cycle or premature aging. The conversion of testosterone into estrogen can repeat plenty of times, and this can keep the estrogen level quite high. The fat tissue can also keep this level high, so the excess fat loss may not be recommended for some ladies, as it can reduce the estrogen level.

Let's get some facts straight! There are also some downsides to this method, and you can discover them below:

- If you want to get all the macronutrients you need for your body, then this method is definitely not for you. One meal will simply not provide you with the nutrient intake you need for the whole day, so you can't expect to have the right ratio of fats, proteins, or carbs that will last you for a day.
- This method is perhaps the most restrictive when it comes to timing (out of the daily fasting methods). Therefore you are being forced to eat all the calories you need in one meal (this may be too much for some people to process).
- There are higher chances of feeling hungry or sick during this program.
- You might be tempted to have food in excess at the only meal you are having during the day. You don't have to eat for three meals when you are having the only meal of the day.

-

Eat Stop Eat Diet

Developed by Brad Pilon, this method involves just one full day of fasting during a week. This process doesn't happen on a daily basis anymore, it happens only on a weekly basis, and it was extended from 16-20 hours to 24 hours. Some people see this method as the easiest one out there, the starting point for Intermittent Fasting. The rules are pretty simple: apply fasting only one day per week, so don't eat anything for 24 hours. You are only allowed to consume water, and nothing else that involves calories. So, no fruits, veggies, juices, or anything like that. Perhaps the only other thing you are allowed to consume is coffee, although it's highly recommended not to use any sugar, milk or cream in it.

However, this is the fasting period. But what about the regular feeding periods? There are no special requirements, in this case, you can still have three meals per day, but you should try to eat healthy food, with fewer calories and carbs. It goes without saying that junk-food, soft drinks, chips, and sweets should be avoided most of the time. Since you are having only one day of fasting, why not take advantage of the fasted state it provides? This is why it's highly recommended to work out during this day, as the fat burning process will be more effective if you are training on this day.

The Alternate-Day Fast

Have you already tried the Eat Stop Eat program, also known as the 24 hours fast? If avoiding anything to eat for 24 hours was a "walk in the park" for you, then you need to try a longer period of fasting. So, here's an interesting program for you! The Alternate-Day Fast was developed by Dr. James B. Johnson (that's right, a doctor, so this should tell you that this program is very legit), and it involves a 12-hour feeding window, followed by a 36-hour fasting period. This program was designed to increase the effects of Intermittent Fasting, as it now brings the fasted state to 24 hours.

The main idea behind it is simple: the longer you fast, the more fat you will burn. Everything makes sense, and the program is totally doable since it was created by a nutritionist. The good doctor has created a few simple rules you will need to follow when applying for this program:

- Respect for the fasting period of 36 hours.

- You can eat as normal as possible during the feeding window.
- You can eat anything you want, but you will still need to avoid excesses. Therefore, you shouldn't eat foods considered "caloric bombs."

If you want to use this method of Intermittent Fasting, then you will need to set up a few things:

- Establish when you want to have the feeding period. For this program, most specialists would agree that it's important to start your feeding window as early in the morning as possible. For example, you can have your first meal at 8 AM and your last meal at 8 PM on a Monday. This should give you plenty of time to have three meals during that day, and perhaps even some snacks. So nothing out of the ordinary, just try not to overeat excessively.
- Your last meal will be followed by a 36-hour fast period. Therefore, if we take the same example, when you have the last meal at 8 PM on a Monday evening, this means that you now start 36 hours of fasting. So you have the rest of the day and the whole next day as a fasting

period. Your next meal will be on Wednesday morning at 8 AM. You can fast more than once per week if you want to maximize the fat-burning process.

Even the creator of this program agrees that not eating anything for about 36 hours can be pretty radical. Therefore the program allows a very small calorie intake during the fasting period. This should represent 20% of your calorie intake from a regular feeding day.

Some of the main benefits of this program can be seen below:

- There are no restrictions in terms of food, but as always, there are some highly recommended food types and ones that should be avoided.
- The method seems to be easy to stick to it and simple as well.
- Deprivation is not something you need to worry about (unlike other diets).
- This program is legit, as it was created by a real doctor (who specialized in nutrition), not a fitness enthusiast or bodybuilder (like other Intermittent Fasting programs).
- Asthma is just one of the conditions this method can improve.

- Just think of the effects this method has on improving your metabolism and extending your lifespan.

Before even thinking of trying an IF program, you will need to know the downsides of it:

- You might experience dizziness, fatigue, or hunger when you try this method for the first few times.
- There is no mention of physical exercise in this method, probably because the plan wants to be regarded as very effective when it comes to burning fat.
- This program is definitely not for anyone with an eating disorder.

Water Fasting

This method is, without a doubt, the most radical and difficult method of fasting, as it involves eliminating any calories from your daily diet. You are only allowed to drink water, so you can't consume anything that has calories, not even an innocent fresh-squeezed juice. Water is good for calming your thirst and to refresh you, but it simply can't be considered a valid source of minerals and vitamins. Your body needs nutrients, but also minerals and vitamins, so it simply can't live on just water. This is why the method is not recommended for a very long time unless you are obese, and nothing else works for you. Still, when you plan to try water fasting for a longer period of time, you can only do it under the supervision of a doctor, as he has to monitor the function of your body and your internal organs.

The record for water fasting was set by a man who managed to fast for more than a year, only drinking water. During this period, he lost 276 pounds (he was literally obese), so this program really worked wonders for him. Most people are capable of water fasting for about a week, but you shouldn't try this method for more than a week. You will need to deal with hunger, dizziness, headaches, and other possible side effects. Plus, it's not very helpful for you if you are also working out. You will feel powerless, and you will feel like you don't have any strength in you. Working out will not be too effective, so you need to set the right expectations when doing this procedure. Don't expect to lose 20 pounds per week! This will most likely not happen.

The water fasting procedure is the "purest" way of fasting and has all the benefits of Intermittent Fasting, plus all its downsides as well. Taking this into account, there are people thinking of trying water fasting for a week a few times per year. The self-cleansing process seems to be working like a charm for this program.

Self-discipline and Technology

Following one of the methods mentioned above may be really tricky, so in order to plan your meals properly, you may need the help of technology. Your smartphone can be used not just for pics and social media; it can be used for planning your meals as well through its calendar. But that's not all! You can also set your daily menu and count the calories you have burned through your daily exercise routine. This can help you set new goals in order to lose more weight and to look great.

When you are on a daily fasting program, you will need to get rid of at least one meal during your day. If you want to achieve more, to burn more fat, then it's highly recommended to get rid of your breakfast. This may sound a bit harsh, but you have no choice. An 8-hour feeding window (or less) is simply not enough to have three whole meals. You might be saying: "But breakfast is the most important meal of the day! It's necessary to get me started for the whole day."

Well, this is a myth that's about to get busted. When you are on a daily Intermittent Fasting program, then you will need to have at least 16 hours of fast. If you schedule your meals properly, most of this period will be overnight when you are at sleep, so you will not be awake to "harass" your refrigerator. When you enter the fast state (after 12 hours from your dinner), it will be very early in the morning, but your body will start to run on fats. This is the right moment to work out and burn fat. Doing your daily exercise on an empty stomach will always have better results for your fat-burning process.

As much as we like to feel that food energizes us, this is wrong. Eating food will provide us the energy source, but not the energy itself. This can only be released through physical exercise. There are only a few people who understand this fact. Otherwise, we would be seeing more people jogging in the morning and more people in the gyms. When you are on a daily fasting program, it's important not to wait too late to have your last meal. Bear in mind that you shouldn't have anything to eat after 6 PM (let's say 8 PM if you prefer). The general rule of thumb is to avoid eating before you sleep. This is why you still need to have 3 hours left from your last meal until you go to bed.

We all like to think that Intermittent Fasting is a way of life, not a diet. There aren't any specific requirements when it comes to the food we eat, so these programs should allow you to eat anything you want, but less of it, since you are concentrating your food into 1-2 meals during the day. If you want to have better results and to speed up the process of fat burning, understanding the nutrition will play a crucial role for you. The most "sinful" types of food are the ones with a high concentration of carbs. These include processed food, but also rice, potatoes, burgers, pizza, bread, pasta, pastries, and many more. Instead of having all of these, you will need to focus on consuming high fiber vegetables and fruits. We all like to eat French fries or rice, but perhaps we need to replace these side dishes and try some vegetables instead. Let's try to avoid high cholesterol food as well, so instead of having some meat fried in cooking oil, let's grill it without using any oil.

Intermittent fasting pushes us to be more disciplined with the food we eat, as it changes our eating habits, not just when we eat but also what we eat. This is why you need to stick to it for as long as possible. Skipping one meal per day is something that all of us can do, so it doesn't require a superhuman effort to follow such a program.

Chapter 9:

Autophagy Is the Possible New "Achilles Heel" Against Cancer

Many specialists see autophagy as a tumor-suppression mechanism. This opinion resulted from early reports proving that the autophagy gene ATG6/BECN1 was monoallelically lost in 40% to 75% of human breast, ovarian, or prostate cancers. Autophagy suppression encourages cancer cell growth, whilst BECN1 heterozygous mutant mice tend to develop lung and liver tumors and lymphomas with long latency. On the other hand, liver-specific or mosaic autophagy deficiency resulted from eliminating the essential autophagy genes ATG5 or ATG7 in mice, which led solely to the production of benign liver tumors. Such discoveries questioned the whole role of autophagy in tumor suppression in the tissues of organs other than the liver, or whether the role of BECN1 in other forms of cancer can be autophagy-related.

Whether BECN1 is a tumor suppressor gene is only based on the allelic loss, and it's often mistaken due to its place adjacent to ovarian and breast tumor suppressor, BRCA1, on human chromosome 17q21. Any mutations suffered in BRCA1 can easily be considered drivers of ovarian and breast cancers. On top of that, hereditary ovarian and breast cancer can appear from different mutations in BRCA1, along with the loss of wild-type allele that may or may not include the elimination of BECN1. Studies conducted on mice have discovered some genetically engineered mouse models (GEMMs) for allelic loss of BECN1 and hereditary breast cancer, which encourage the activation of p53 and can lower tumorigenesis, which happens to be the exact opposite result expected if BECN1 was acting as a tumor suppressor.

Different mutations in BECN1 were evaluated in tumor sequencing data from 10,000 subjects with tumors with matched tissue in the Cancer Genome Atlas as well as other databases. Large eliminations of both BECN1 and BRCA1 as well as eliminations of just BRCA1 (and not BECN1) could be found in ovarian and breast cancers, meaning that the loss of BRCA1 was the driving mutation in these types of cancer. The loss of BECN1 in any form of human cancer can't be disconnected from the loss of BRCA1, meaning that BECN1 can't be considered a tumor suppressor in most human cancers.

That said, autophagy deficiency can lead to oxidative stress as well as to the activation of the DNA damage response and genome instability, which is considered a known cause of cancer inception and progression. Increased oxidative stress can trigger the master regulator of nuclear factor, antioxidant defense, and also NRF2, which is considered a tumor growth stimulator. Autophagy failure in the liver is toxic, and it can lead to inflammation and chronic cell death of hepatocytes, all of which are also known for being drivers of liver cancer. When p62 is deficient, it can lower toxicity and tumorigenesis caused by a defective autophagy process. However, when p62 is properly expressed, it can encourage tumor growth and oxidative stress along with regulating oncogenic pathways, especially those involving mTOR, NRF2, or NF-kB.

Autophagy can also be seen as a tumor promoter. Cancer cells can be dependent on autophagy, probably more than other normal tissues or cells. This situation is caused by deficiencies in the microenvironment, but also by enhanced biosynthetic and metabolic demands imposed by uncontrolled proliferation. Basal autophagy can be upregulated in hypoxic tumor regions, exactly where it's very important for tumor cell survival. Autophagy can also be upregulated in RAS-transformed cancer cells, and it can encourage their growth, survival, as well as tumorigenesis, invasion, and metastasis. The susceptibility to stress or the mitochondrial metabolic defects from autophagy deficiency in RAS-driven cancers is involved in this mechanism. This is why RAS-driven cancers may be dependent on autophagy.

Other studies have shown that a deficiency in ATG17/FIP200 can constrain the growth of mammary cancers in mice. This emphasizes the role that autophagy has in promoting tumorigenesis and how applicable the whole concept of autophagy dependency is in cancer.

Chapter 10:

Autophagy and Its Great Success

Some of the significant benefits of Autophagy are reflected in the general health of your body. There is still a lot to be learned about Autophagy, but we know for a fact what some of the major benefits of it are for your health. There are plenty of illnesses you can get from eating on a "standard diet" like diabetes, heart, liver, or kidney diseases. Luckily for us, there are some methods we can use to treat or prevent them that we don't even know about. No, it's not about medical treatment, not about medication, just simple procedures we can do on our bodies to help stop, prevent, or reverse these diseases.

Autophagy can have a major impact on certain diseases or conditions like:

- Alzheimer's Disease
- Parkinson's Disease
- Osteoporosis
- Diabetes
- Cancer

We will start with one illness or condition at a time, so we can go through them in-depth.

Alzheimer's Disease.

As you probably know, Alzheimer's Disease is a neurodegenerative condition; this means that damage to brain cells can cause this situation. Autophagy represents the method that brain cells use to get rid of damaged structures inside the cells, including the ones impaired in Alzheimer's disease. Brain cells can, at times, incorrectly produce a toxic form of amyloid-beta peptide, which is nothing more than a toxic protein that can cause AD. Autophagy can track down amyloids and eliminate them in different types of brain cells.

When the amyloid-beta peptide is accumulating in your brain cells, it can be considered a major signal for AD. So far, countless therapies have been tried in an attempt to cure Alzheimer's Disease, but all of them failed, as none of those therapies managed to track down the root of the disease and eliminate it. AD can be considered a neurodegenerative condition caused by imbalanced protein degradation or production. By increasing the protein degradation capacity of the neuron, the amyloid load will be reduced along with the cellular dysfunction and the amyloid-induced inflammation.

Autophagy can provide the solution for this problem, as it represents a "self-eating" pathway specialized in eliminating toxic or damaged proteins from your brain cells. During AD pathogenesis, it is easy to observe an impairment of Autophagy. Although this has been tested on mice, there isn't any reason why it shouldn't be the case in humans. The transgenic mouse model systems can show high or low levels of Autophagy, and they can also be used to investigate how the autophagy machinery is capable of regulating and recognizing amyloid metabolism in neurons or microglial cells in the brain. Also, this model can be used to discover whether upregulating Autophagy can be useful for restoring cognitive functions in AD. Studies are still being conducted on this matter, and the results will be revealed soon enough. However, it's fair to conclude that Autophagy can play a major role in preventing, stopping, and possibly reversing Alzheimer's Disease (AD).

There are also studies confirming that people with type 2 diabetes have a higher risk of Alzheimer's disease (about 50-60% higher).

However, Autophagy induced through fasting can help you solve this problem:

- It can clear the beta-amyloid plaques that are starting to accumulate with Alzheimer's progression and cognitive decline. As it turns out, Alzheimer's is also linked with insulin resistance and obesity.
- Ketone bodies like beta-hydroxybutyrate can block the part of the immune system responsible for regulating inflammatory diseases like Alzheimer's or arthritis.
- Ketone bodies can also increase BDNF (brain-derived neurotrophic factor) and decrease oxidative stress. They can also lower the excitement in your brain caused by excess glutamate or lack of GABA (Gamma-aminobutyric acid).

The fasted state, when ketone levels are higher, can also sharpen your mind and can prevent it from becoming dull due to mild stress response. The fasting process can also seriously boost your brain performance, and there are plenty of people who claim that they've experienced an enhanced sense of awareness, mental clarity, focus, motivation, and attention. This can only be the result of an increase in BDNF or other neurotrophic factors/hormones like cortisol, norepinephrine, adrenaline, or other endorphins.

Parkinson's Disease

Most of the principles and tests from Alzheimer's Disease can also apply to Parkinson's Disease (PD). In fact, most specialists would like to consider the benefits of Autophagy on both of these neurodegenerative diseases, and not to take them separately. Just like in the case of Alzheimer's Disease, for this illness, many studies have been conducted to discover the role played by Autophagy and how it can influence this condition.

Did you know that Parkinson's Disease is the second most common neurodegenerative disease, and in most cases, this illness is sporadic and is only inherited in 5% of cases? PD genes include:

a) SNCA is a gene encoding alpha-synuclein, the main component of the Lewy bodies that accumulate in the brain of patients.
b) LRRK2 encodes a huge multi-domain protein. Variable LRRK2 mutants are responsible for more than 10% of familial

and 3% of sporadic Parkinson's Disease cases.
c) PINK1 and Parkin represent genes involved in mitochondrial maintenance and turnover. Mutations in these genes are usually associated with early-onset PD.
d) DJ-1 protein, mutations in which are responsible for 1-2 % of autosomal recessive PD.

As it turns out, autophagy defects can be involved in PD pathogenesis. Parkinson's Disease-related VPS35 AND D620N mutants can constrain Autophagy and can seriously impair the trafficking of the autophagy protein ATG9A. But that's not all! Aberrant autophagy activity has already been discovered in Parkinson's Disease patients diagnosed with substantia nigra (SN) defects. Therefore, these are the effects improper Autophagy has on people suffering from this illness.

Moving on to more positive effects, it looks like inducing Autophagy by manipulating the Polo-like kinase 2, or just activating chaperone-mediated Autophagy can decrease alpha-synuclein aggregation.

Osteoporosis

As you probably know, osteoporosis is a bone disease caused by too much bone loss. This can lead to bones being weak and breaking very easily from a variety of causes. Literally, osteoporosis means "porous bone." This condition usually occurs in seniors, but it can also happen to normal adults or even children.

Since the development of studies on Autophagy, it has been proven that this process has a key role in maintaining bone homeostasis. Multiple studies (especially *in vitro* ones) have clearly proven that pharmacological inhibition of Autophagy in different osteoblast environments can lead to higher oxidative stress and can encourage apoptosis in these cells. On the other hand, initializing Autophagy in these osteoblast cells can constrain apoptosis and lower oxidative stress. Speaking of inhibitors, estrogen can also discourage any osteoblast apoptosis *in vitro*, triggering Autophagy in these cells.

No one can doubt the role of Autophagy when osteoblasts are being added into the bone matrix and transformed into osteocytes. During this transition, osteoblasts can suffer obvious shape changes, correlated with a serious decrease in the number (and size) of organelles.

We can only assume that there is an increase in Autophagy taking place during the transition from osteoblasts to osteocytes. Such an increase is caused by the need for nutrient preservation and faster recycling of the organelles. In the meantime, the cell is experiencing actin-rich prolongations, and it can easily adapt to any type of environment affected by hypoxia. As it turns out, LC3 is expressed more effectively in osteocytes than in osteoblasts.

I like to think of osteocytes as cells that can be found in spaces delimited by mineralized bone matrix, and this environment is more affected by accumulated oxidative stress and hypoxia. In these conditions, guess what will determine the survival of osteocytes? Yep, you've guessed it! It's Autophagy. Osteocytes have a higher autophagic activity after going through hypoxia and nutrient deprivation *in vitro*, which are very similar conditions to the ones found in osteocytes *in vivo*.

On top of that, as a response to calcium-mediated stress, the activity of hypoxia-inducing transcription factor (also known as HIF-1) can make a positive adjustment to Autophagy, proving that low oxygen tension can act as an autophagy regulator in this cell type. Autophagy in osteocytes can be induced by a low-dose glucocorticoid treatment as a response to higher oxidative stress caused by treatment, saving the viability of these cells.

There are also other studies that emphasize the role of Autophagy in bone resorption by osteoclasts. Also, as it turns out, proteins implicated in the autophagic pathway can play an essential role in regulating osteoclastogenesis, proving that this process is involved both in bone resorption and formation. Bafilomycin, which is an autophagy inhibitor, can contribute to decreasing the resorptive activity.

Studies conducted in mice (with results that are applicable for humans as well) have shown that a mutation in the gene encoding the p62 protein can result in a phenotype very similar to Paget's disease of bone. This condition is characterized by an excessive increase in bone remodeling and vulnerability to fractures. Autophagy levels can become elevated during osteoclastogenesis under conditions of higher oxidative stress (caused by glucocorticoid treatment) and hypoxia. In this situation, Autophagy can have a protective role by lowering cell stress and increasing the viability and formation of osteoclasts.

The elimination of genes encoding key proteins involved in the formation of the autophagosome (LC3, ATG5, ATG7, ATG4B) can cause serious changes to the brush border of osteoclasts, and therefore, it can lower bone resorption and enhance bone volume. This can prevent bone loss in mice following an ovariectomy procedure. There are some specialists who believe that suppressing Autophagy in osteoclasts can be seen as a therapeutic mechanism against bone diseases, at least in cases when there is too much increase in bone resorption. At least on mice, genetic and pharmacological suppression of Autophagy can lead to lower bone resorption and osteoclastogenesis, discouraging any bone loss due to glucocorticoid treatment or ovariectomy.

More recent studies have shown that Autophagy can be regarded as an important factor in the bone growth process. Autophagy can regulate the secretion of type II collagen by chondrocytes of the epiphyseal disc, and all of this is done through the influence of FGF18. However, the mechanisms that allow Autophagy to regulate the secretion of collagen are not yet fully understood.

There are so many things yet to be discovered about Autophagy, but some of the discoveries already made can shock you. For instance, there was a study conducted over 618 adult Chinese subjects that proved the role of expressing genes that regulate the autophagic pathway in influencing the height and stature variation of individuals. If we just think that Autophagy enhances the viability of chondrocytes, we can easily add this feature to the protective role that Autophagy can have over these cells in the epiphyseal disc, thus having a major impact over the growth of long bones.

Have you ever wondered what exactly happens internally when you fracture a bone? Apparently, in this case, Autophagy can be triggered to repair the bone after it has been fractured. In this case, autophagy functions as a defense mechanism (against cell stress) triggered by nutrient deprivation (interruption or reduction), which followed the bone fracture. Therefore, Autophagy can have a lot to say in bone tissue homeostasis.

More recent studies have proven that genetic and chloroquine autophagy inhibition via the selective elimination of the ATG7 gene in monocytes can lower osteoclastogenesis, and it can also reduce bone loss in animal models. If you administer an antibody against sclerostin, which is a known suppressor of bone formation by osteoblasts, you will notice that it can prevent any bone loss caused by glucocorticoid treatment in male mice. The study showed how great quantities of glucocorticoid treatment lowered the percentage of LC3-positive osteoblasts (which is known as an autophagic marker) and also decreased the viability of these cells, leading to bone loss. On the other hand, if you choose to treat the mice with the anti-sclerostin antibody, you will notice how it maintains the viability of osteoblasts by improving Autophagy in these cells and reducing the bone loss caused by glucocorticoid treatment. More studies are required to find out why these mechanisms and treatments (sclerostin and its antibody) can regulate the autophagic pathway in bone cells.

Without a doubt, Autophagy can maintain bone mass while maintaining the viability of osteoblasts. Based on this idea, if you eliminate the FIP200 gene (which is very important in autophagosome formation) from osteoblasts, this can lead to osteopenia in rats, caused by reducing the bone formation process in these cells.

If you choose to eliminate the ATG7 gene (important for inducing Autophagy) from osteocytes, it can lead to a decrease in the bone mass of 6-month-old male or female mice, similar to natural aging. Another study shows a connection between the lowered autophagic activity in osteocytes and the bone loss process during aging for senile rats. The same result was achieved after rapamycin (known for inducing Autophagy as well) has decreased osteoporosis by triggering Autophagy in osteocytes.

Apparently, there is a relation between the mechanism used by Autophagy to reduce bone loss caused by aging and the antioxidant effect of Autophagy on these bone cells. Higher oxidative stress in the knockout animal models can only support this hypothesis.

If we think of estrogen deficiency, this is normally considered the most important cause of bone loss for women during the postmenopausal phase. As it turns out, higher oxidative stress applied to the bone tissue represents one of the main factors that determine bone loss during aging.

In other words, decreasing the autophagic process can lead to higher oxidative stress, and this will eventually cause bone loss. An increase in the autophagic pathway can have the opposite effect, so it can promote lower oxidative stress and can prevent bone loss. Such a hypothesis correlates the level of Autophagy in osteocytes with the oxidative stress and bone loss caused by estrogen deficiency noticed in the tibia of ovariectomized rats.

Numerous studies in animal and *in vitro* models support a possible connection between autophagic dysfunction and osteoporosis. This connection has not yet been studied in humans, but there is genetic screening research that shows a direct relationship between the expression of the autophagic pathway and variation in bone mineral density. The study was conducted on 984 individuals, so it's pretty conclusive. The researchers agreed that there might be an implication of the autophagic pathway in the development of osteoporosis.

Other preclinical *in vivo* and *in vitro* studies demonstrate a connection between osteoporosis and the deregulation of the autophagic pathway.

Diabetes

Autophagy is becoming a very popular and interesting topic lately; this is why more scientists are curious about it and are conducting studies on this topic. The main reason why it's becoming so popular is the impact it has on your health, particularly in this case, the impact it has on diabetes.

A recent study proved that cyclical fasting could lead to the repair of beta cells in mouse models of type 1 diabetes. Autophagy is usually followed by a massive boost of stem cells, which usually replenishes or repairs the beta cells affected by the autoimmune processes. Now, I know what you are thinking! These studies are conducted on mice and rats; they can't apply to humans. Well, before you jump to conclusions, try to read the following lines.

Another study showed the effects following a keto diet has on type 2 diabetes (it can significantly lower its risk). This time, we are talking about studies on humans.

The main idea behind the benefits of Autophagy in diabetes management is simple. Autophagy is usually triggered after 24 hours of fasting when the glucose and blood sugar levels are very low. As it's a phase of Intermittent Fasting, and it can also be induced through the keto diet, Autophagy sums up the benefits from both of these procedures, including the positive effect it has on diabetes. By the time it reaches the autophagy phase, your body is already running smoothly on fats, which means that your glucose reserves are getting lower. This process will eventually activate insulin (as it's getting lower and lower), and insulin is known to regulate the blood sugar level. Lower glucose and blood sugar level means reversing the prediabetes condition or even diabetes itself, assuming the disease is not so serious that it requires insulin administration.

The keto diet does the same thing as Intermittent Fasting; the only difference is that one program requires you to eat only during a feeding window, while the other one is more about the food you eat (fatty food choices) and less about starvation. Your body will be fully prepared to run on fats since the keto diet gets your body into the metabolic state of ketosis. During this phase, the liver releases chemical compounds called ketones, responsible for breaking down the fat tissue and releasing the energy stored in there. Glucose deprivation will simply prevent your body from running on glucose again and prevent it from being stored in your body and blood. In these conditions, you would expect the insulin to regulate the blood sugar level with increasing effectiveness, until it reaches a decent level and you are no longer in a diabetic (or prediabetic) condition.

Cancer

Cancer is one of the deadliest diseases known to man, and the number of cancer cases in the population has been increasing very rapidly. It can affect most of your internal organs, and in many cases, it can't be detected until later phases. A simple cause of cancer would be accumulated damage to your genes. Your lifestyle can significantly increase the risk of cancer, but there are also some other external causes. Although cancer can be caused by external factors like exposure to different chemicals, UV radiation, radioactive materials, and so on, let's face it, the majority of cancers are caused by lifestyle factors. These could be smoking, drinking alcohol, or some toxic chemicals found in the food we eat.

When we say that cancer is caused by accumulated damage to the genes, we mean, in fact, damage to the cells. As you already know by now, Autophagy is considered an intracellular "housekeeper," meaning it cleans up the mess inside your cells. By mess, we mean old and damaged cell parts like organelles, proteins, or cell tissues. Since this process is about covering the mess in a membrane and eating it up, you can imagine that there are no damaged or "broken" parts left.

A proper autophagy process will clean up everything there is to clean at an intracellular level. We are talking about repairing, replenishing or replacing these cell parts, so picture Autophagy as the best "mechanic" out there and the cell as a car. Everything will function properly after Autophagy is finished with the cell. If you induce Autophagy more often, the process will not allow cancer to begin in any cell in your body. This is why it not only has a spectacular anti-aging effect, but it also has an impressive effect on cancer. Of course, you can't expect Autophagy to cure anyone of cancer when they are in metastasis. However, if you manage to induce Autophagy, this process can significantly lower the risk of cancer. Some people who are fully aware of this benefit are inducing Autophagy a few times per year. There is nothing like a good clean up a few times per year.

Most specialists regard Autophagy is the cellular process that breaks down cells for later reuse. It's crucial for proper cell function and for protecting the cells of your body, and this may be the reason that Autophagy plays a major role in preventing and treating cancer. If you are following chemotherapy, Intermittent Fasting can reduce nausea and headaches caused by your chemotherapy treatment.

There are several studies proving that Autophagy can increase the effectiveness of tumor-suppressing genes. Lower Autophagy may help with tumor formation, but it can't be considered the only one cause responsible for the spread or growth of a malignant tumor.

If you want to find out more effects that Autophagy can have on the quality of life during chemotherapy, take a look below:

- It encourages cellular regeneration.
- It defends your blood against the harmful effects of chemotherapy.
- It can decrease the impact of side effects like headaches, fatigue, nausea, and cramps.

Apparently, Intermittent Fasting can seriously improve the quality of life during chemotherapy for women suffering from ovarian or breast cancer by giving them more energy, a higher tolerance to side effects, and higher tolerance to chemotherapy itself.

Conclusion

As much as we hate to admit it, we live in a sick society where most people are struggling with diseases and medical conditions, many of which are caused by the food we eat. High-quality food is not easily accessible, and many people can't afford it. Somehow supermarkets are all full of processed food, and this is what causes most of the problems we have with health today. Every company working in the food processing industry has renounced any principles regarding quality and instead focuses on making massive quantities to maximize their profits. Let's face it! Authorities are too permissive with the food or drinks that are allowed to be sold in supermarkets or even restaurants.

It looks like we are now experiencing a huge problem in nutrition, as most of the food we consume is very rich in carbs and sugar. The last component can be held responsible for most deaths in recent years, more than any other substance abuse. Sugar is the poison we consume on a daily basis, and it looks like we simply can't help it. We can't resist or stay away from it, and on top of that, we even feed it to our children. Most of the diseases and conditions we know today are caused by the abuse of carbs and sugar. Let's enumerate just a few of them: diabetes; heart, liver, kidney and lung diseases; Parkinson's and Alzheimer's Disease; and many types of cancer.

It looks like medicine is not advanced enough to deal with all these problems. If, in the past, you could die from pneumonia or tuberculosis, nowadays, the most common ways to dye are of a heart attack, cancer (for most internal organs), or other serious diseases. It looks like we never learn our lesson, although we know exactly what can cause these issues, we keep on consuming the same food, as we somehow find it very tasty. Health services are becoming more expensive, as the health system has to deal with plenty of dangerous diseases, and it looks like they're spreading like wildfire.

Truth be told, the development of these diseases is encouraged by the modern times we are living in. We are experiencing plenty of stress, we are too sedentary, and we don't indulge in enough physical activities. It looks like our whole universe is on our tablet or smartphone, as we can barely remove our eyes from them. Instead of working out, we prefer to spend our time on social media on these devices. We don't have enough time to cook, and we are always time-restricted. We are forced to do as many tasks as possible in a very limited period of time. This is where the stress comes from. It can be job-related, or it can be debt-related. Every one of us is exposed to these two types of stress. Stress can cause compulsive eating, and guess what we eat when we are stressed? Carbs!

The immune system of our body is seriously challenged by all the illnesses and conditions we are experiencing today. Unfortunately, it's also weakened since we don't allow it to fight against them, we constantly take pills, and while they can mask the symptoms, they are affecting our immune system in the long run. Luckily for us, our body can provide solutions for the health problems we are experiencing.

Autophagy is one of the most beneficial processes that can be performed by our bodies. It manifests at an intracellular level and is known for repairing, recycling, or replacing old and damaged cell parts like organelles, proteins, or cell tissues. Now, this may not sound too interesting, but that's where the magic happens. The intracellular level plays a very crucial role in preventing, stopping, or even reversing some of the most important diseases we are experiencing today. Autophagy is decisive for curing or stopping these diseases as well as for the anti-aging process and for weight loss.

There are three types of Autophagy: macroautophagy, microautophagy, and chaperone-mediated Autophagy. It all sounds very interesting, but it's not that easy to induce Autophagy. This process can be triggered by nutrient deprivation or by really intense training. Therefore, Autophagy can be activated through Intermittent Fasting or through a keto diet. The first method involves dividing your time into a fasting and feeding period, making the fasting period a lot longer than the feeding window if we are talking about daily fasting. It's a process of self-discipline and restricting yourself to eat only during the feeding window. Autophagy can be triggered after 24 hours of fasting (meaning 24 hours since your last meal). This requires no calorie consumption in the fasting period unless you are following a certain type of Intermittent Fasting program.

The keto diet is a very popular form of LCHF (low carbs high fats) diet, which aims to induce the metabolic state of ketosis in which ketones are released to break down fat tissue. Both of these procedures (Intermittent Fasting and the keto diet) are known for enabling the body to run on fats. This is why the keto diet is a glucose deprivation program, as it stops feeding your body with glucose, and it replaces it with fats. When you feed your body with fats, it will run on fats, so it will burn a lot of them. If you also exercise, then it will burn the fat you eat as well as your fat reserves.

Breaking down the fat reserves will release the energy stored in there along with the toxins protected by the fat tissue, so it has a double advantage (fat loss and detox). Autophagy can also be triggered by very intense sessions of training, like HIIT (High-Intensity Interval Training), the type of endurance training that can apply enough stress at the intracellular level to trigger Autophagy.

There are a few programs for Intermittent Fasting, and there isn't such a thing as an ideal program, as it depends more on the characteristics of each individual and what he is trying to achieve. Some people would insist that daily fasting is better; others insist on fasting for a longer period. Most fasting programs should be associated with an LCHF diet and physical exercise. This is how you can maximize the effect of this procedure, whether you aim to cause more fat loss or to Induce Autophagy.

When it comes to the keto diet, having some knowledge about the food groups will help you a lot, as you will know for sure which food types have a higher ratio of carbs and which don't. Hint: you might completely eliminate or significantly reduce the consumption of burgers,